Haemodynamic Monitoring and Manipulation

An easy learning guide

Easy Learning Guides from M&K

The array of complex functions carried out by senior clinical staff can be quite bewildering to more junior staff. Some of them would like to wave a magic wand that makes them instantly knowledgeable and confident. These *Easy Learning Guides* are not a magic wand, but they are probably the next best thing! They were written by a health professional who had to learn by experience, along with everyone else, but who knows that there are far easier ways to pick up these essential skills.

These no-fuss practical guides promote confidence and competence in several key areas of clinical practice, including:

Artificial Ventilation

Arterial Blood Gas Analysis

Cardiac Arrhythmia Recognition

Fluid & Electrolyte Balance & Control

Neurological Observations & Their Significance

To find out more about these and other books published by M&K, as well as their wide range of clinical training courses, visit:

www.mkupdate.co.uk

Haemodynamic Monitoring and Manipulation

An easy learning guide

Fiona Foxall MA, RGN, ENB100, DPSN, BSc, PGCE

Head of Division, Continuing Development,
School of Health, University of Wolverhampton,
West Midlands, UK

With original artwork by Helen Blackburn

Haemodynamic Monitoring and Manipulation:
An Easy Learning Guide
Fiona Foxall

ISBN: 978-1-905539-46-8

First published 2009

British Library Catalogue in Publication Data
A catalogue record for this book is available from the British Library

Notice:
Clinical practice and medical knowledge constantly evolve. Standard safety precautions must be followed, but, as knowledge is broadened by research, changes in practice, treatment and drug therapy may become necessary or appropriate. Readers must check the most current product information provided by the manufacturer of each drug to be administered and verify the dosages and correct administration, as well as contraindications. It is the responsibility of the practitioner, utilising the experience and knowledge of the patient, to determine dosages and the best treatment for each individual patient. Any brands mentioned in this book are as examples only and are not endorsed by the Publisher. Neither the Publisher nor the author assume any liability for any injury and/or damage to persons or property arising from this publication.

The Publisher
To contact M&K Publishing write to:
M&K Update Ltd · The Old Bakery · St. John's Street
Keswick · Cumbria CA12 5AS
Tel: 01768 773030 · Fax: 01768 781099
publishing@mkupdate.co.uk
www.mkupdate.co.uk

Designed and typeset in Adobe Garamond 10/12 by S. Maria Hampshire.
Cover design by Luke Kelsey.

Printed in England by Reeds Printers, Penrith, Cumbria.

DEDICATION

For Peter:

Sleep peacefully my darling.

Contents

Acknowledgements

Thanks, as always, to Chris, Helen and Matthew Blackburn for all their help and support.

Introduction

The adequacy of the cardiorespiratory system can generally be gauged from basic clinical signs such as heart rate, blood pressure, respiratory rate and depth, skin texture and colour, use of accessory muscles of respiration and mental status. These basic signs should never be ignored, but in critical illness, basic clinical assessment alone may be unreliable and misleading. Therefore further monitoring techniques are usually required.

Appropriate haemodynamic monitoring is essential when caring for the critically ill patient, because it provides very valuable information about the circulatory status of the patient. It aids in early detection of shock and precise diagnosis, guides therapy, and monitors the effects of therapy. Cardiac output and the circulation can be manipulated by fluid and drug administration to ensure good oxygen delivery to the tissues but, in order to do this, ongoing monitoring is required (Jevon and Ewens, 2002).

Many healthcare professionals find it difficult to get to grips with the more complex forms of haemodynamic monitoring and the use of inotropic and vasoactive agents; indeed these things can seem rather daunting. If you work your way through this book and carry out the exercises, you will soon become more confident and competent about haemodynamic monitoring and manipulation as well as understanding all the information that initially seems so complicated.

Here's to easy learning!

How to use this workbook

It might sound obvious, but you should start at the beginning. Even if you feel quite happy about haemodynamic monitoring, it will be good revision. Steadily work through the material, ensuring you understand the information in each chapter before moving on to the next. Once you have read each chapter, complete the Consolidation section; these will make sure you understand the information sufficiently. Chapter 7 is a bit different from the other chapters; answer the questions and fill in the gaps as you work through the case studies. It will be helpful if you can find a mentor to discuss anything you are unsure about.

If you don't know a particular answer, try to work it out with the information you have already read. If you still can't, discuss it with your mentor. If it is still unclear, then look up the answer in the Answer section at the back of the book. If you do look up the answer, make sure you *understand* it – don't just accept it. You can talk to your mentor if you have any problems. The Answer section should only be used as a last resort and for checking purposes. It goes without saying that you will learn far more by working things out for yourself than merely reading the explanations provided.

If you already have a reasonable knowledge and understanding of haemodynamic monitoring and manipulation, you could – if you prefer – attempt the Consolidation sections before reading the explanatory text. This will give you a good idea of your current level of knowledge and will also identify any gaps, which you can then concentrate on filling.

Aims of this workbook

This book aims to extend your knowledge and clinical application of haemodynamic monitoring and manipulation.

After completing this workbook you will be able to:

- Discuss the normal physiological mechanisms for maintaining blood pressure.
- State the normal pressures within the cardiovascular system.
- Define and state the significance of each parameter measured during haemodynamic monitoring.
- Discuss monitoring of blood pressure using an arterial line.
- Discuss monitoring and maintenance of central venous pressure.
- Discuss monitoring and maintenance of cardiac output and tissue perfusion.
- Discuss the effects of shock on the cardiovascular system and the pressures within it.
- Discuss how cardiovascular pressures are manipulated by titration of inotropic and vasoactive agents.
- Recognise abnormalities and describe what actions are appropriate.

Chapter 1

Physiological maintenance of blood pressure

The cardiovascular system exists to provide tissue perfusion. Tissue perfusion ensures the body's cells are provided with oxygen and nutrients at the same time as removing metabolic wastes (Gonce-Morton *et al.*, 2005).

What is blood pressure?

All critically ill patients will need to have continuous blood pressure monitoring and you need to understand the significance of abnormal blood pressure. To understand it, you must first understand how normal blood pressure is maintained.

> **Simply, blood pressure is the pressure exerted against the arterial walls during the cardiac cycle.**
> (Gonce-Morton *et al.*, 2005)

Mean arterial pressure is comparable to the perfusion pressure of the aorta, its major branches and major organs throughout the complete cardiac cycle. It is therefore representative of the average arterial pressure present in the peripheral circulation (Viney, 1999).

Controlling blood pressure

There are six physiological mechanisms for controlling blood pressure, namely: maintenance of blood volume, endocrine control, equilibration of cardiac input and output, peripheral resistance, the renin–angiotensin system and the baroreceptor reflex.

1. Maintenance of blood volume

If the fluid volume in the cardiovascular system is reduced, thirst then develops. This makes us take in more fluid. At the same time, urine output reduces as a result of ADH (antidiuretic hormone) production (ADH conserves fluid within the body by stimulating water reabsorption in the nephron). This is summarised in Figs 1.1 and 1.2.

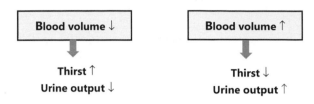

Fig. 1.1 *Maintenance of blood volume.*

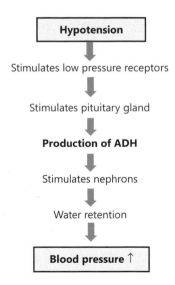

Fig. 1.2 *Production and effects of antidiuretic hormone (ADH).*

Conversely, the fluid volume in the cardiovascular system is increased, thirst is absent and urine output increases to rid the body of excess fluid.

2. Endocrine control

If blood pressure decreases, the adrenal medullae are stimulated to produce adrenaline and noradrenaline, which increase cardiac contractility, which in turn increases cardiac output and therefore blood pressure increases (Fig. 1.3).

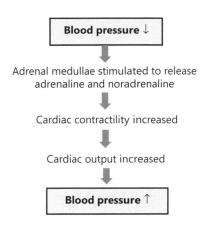

Fig. 1.3 *Mechanisms of endocrine control.*

3. Equilibration of cardiac input and output

To understand this, you will need to understand Starling's Law of the heart.

> **Starling's Law of the heart**
> The force of contraction is proportional
> to the length of the muscle fibres.

This means as the heart fills with increasing volumes of blood, the myocardium is stretched and the ventricles contract more forcefully (Viney, 1999). To put it simply, the end-diastolic length of the myocardial fibres is proportional to the end-diastolic volume. Put even more simply, the more blood that is in the ventricle at the end of diastole, the more the cardiac muscle will stretch. The more cardiac muscle is stretched, the more forcefully it will contract – just like an elastic band! So the heart is able to regulate itself to equilibrate intake and output. Starling's Law is demonstrated when there is a rise in venous pressure.

Rise in venous pressure

If there is an increase in venous return, the amount of blood in the ventricles at the end of diastole will increase. The ventricular muscle will stretch to accommodate the extra volume and will eject blood more forcefully (because the cardiac muscle contracts more forcefully when stretched).

Rise in arterial pressure

If there is an increase in arterial pressure, there will be more resistance to the outflow of blood from the left ventricle. Therefore, cardiac work increases to eject the blood from the left ventricle and output will equate to input.

4. Maintenance of peripheral resistance

Sympathetic nerve impulses maintain a permanent state of partial vasoconstriction – this is known as **sympathetic tone**. Without these sympathetic impulses, blood vessels would be in a constant state of vasodilation and the blood pressure would be too low to sustain life. Sympathetic impulses increase or decrease in response to an increase or decrease in blood pressure (Fig. 1.4).

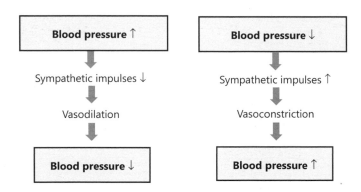

Fig. 1.4 *Sympathetic nerve control.*

5. The renin–angiotensin system

If there is a decrease in arterial pressure, the juxtaglomerular cells in the kidneys are stimulated to produce renin, an enzyme that stimulates the production of angiotensin I from inactive angiotensinogen. Angiotensin I stimulates the production of angiotensin-converting enzyme (ACE) from the liver, which converts angiotensin I to angiotensin II. See Fig. 1.5. Angiotensin II raises blood pressure in *four* ways (Janson-Cohen, 2005):

(i) It increases cardiac output and vasoconstriction.

(ii) It stimulates the adrenal cortex to produce aldosterone (resulting in sodium and water retention which also raises blood pressure).

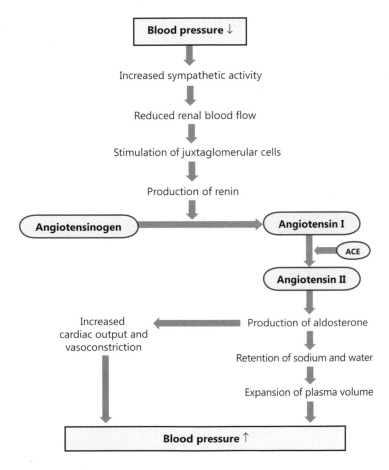

Fig. 1.5 *Renin–angiotensin system (ACE, angiotensin-converting enzyme).*

(iii) It stimulates release of ADH from the pituitary gland (which increases water reabsorption).

(iv) It stimulates the thirst centres in the hypothalamus (increasing fluid consumption).

6. The baroreceptor reflex

Baroreceptors are located in three places (Martini, 2006):

- In the carotid sinuses (the chambers near the bases of the internal carotid arteries of the neck).

- In the aortic sinuses (the pockets in the walls of the ascending aorta adjacent to the heart).

- In the wall of the right atrium.

Changes in blood pressure stimulate the *baroreceptor reflex*, which adjusts the blood pressure to maintain adequate tissue perfusion.

When BP increases

When blood pressure increases there is *increased* baroreceptor activity. This then stimulates the cardiac inhibitory c entre, so reducing sympathetic impulses to the heart and arterioles. This has two major effects:

- Decrease in cardiac output due to inhibition of sympathetic impulses and increasing parasympathetic stimulation.

- Widespread peripheral vasodilation due to inhibition of excitatory neurons in the vasomotor centre.

As a result, BP *reduces* to normal (Martini, 2006). See Fig. 1.6.

When BP decreases

When blood pressure reduces there is *reduced* baroreceptor output. This has two major effects:

- An increase in cardiac output due to stimulation of cardio-acceleratory centres (increasing sympathetic nerve activity to the heart) and inhibition of the cardio-inhibitory centres (reducing parasympathetic activity to the heart).

- Widespread peripheral vasoconstriction which is caused by increased sympathetic activity.

As a result, BP *increases* to normal (Martini, 2006). See Fig. 1.7.

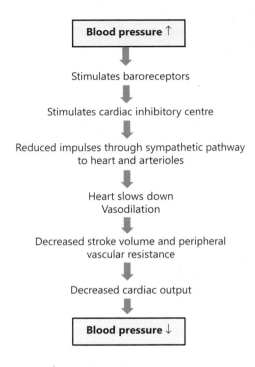

Fig. 1.6 *The baroreceptor reflex in hypertension.*

Effects of hypertension

A sustained blood pressure above 140/90 mmHg is the usual criterion (in adults) for diagnosing hypertension (Martini, 2006). Everyone has transient periods of hypertension at some time or other, for example, when they are anxious or exercising hard, but sustained hypertension has undesirable physiological effects. Hypertension increases oxygen demand on the heart as the left ventricle has to maintain an increased workload to maintain adequate tissue perfusion. If the coronary circulation cannot maintain adequate cardiac perfusion, cardiac ischaemia will result. In addition, hypertension places more stress on the arteriolar walls throughout the body. Treatment is first aimed at the cause of the hypertension, then at the symptoms.

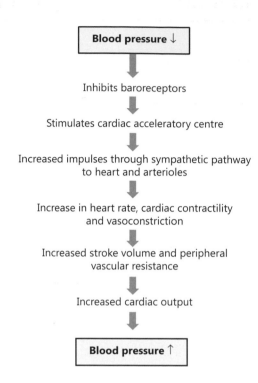

Fig. 1.7 *The baroreceptor reflex in hypotension.*

Effects of hypotension

More commonly in critically ill patients, hypotension occurs as a result of a failing cardiovascular system. This results in reduced tissue perfusion and therefore tissue hypoxia and a build up of waste products. In the critically ill, it is therefore essential to monitor blood pressure closely and to give appropriate and swift treatment to maintain adequate blood pressure.

Consolidation

See pages 113–114 for answers

1.1   How is blood pressure defined?

_____

_____

1.2   Name six natural mechanisms for maintaining blood pressure.

_____

_____

_____

1.3   How is blood volume maintained?

_____

_____

_____

1.4   In what way does the endocrine system help in the control of blood pressure?

_____

_____

_____

1.5   How does the heart equilibrate input and output?

1.6   How is peripheral resistance maintained?

1.7   Describe the renin–angiotensin system.

1.8   Where are baroreceptors located?

1.9   Describe the baroreceptor reflex in hypertension.

1.10   Describe the baroreceptor reflex in hypotension.

_____

_____

_____

1.11   What are the major effects of hypertension?

_____

_____

1.12   What are the major effects of hypotension?

_____

_____

Notes

Chapter 2

Monitoring blood pressure using an arterial line

The most common way of monitoring the blood pressure of the critically ill patient is through the insertion of an arterial line. As well as allowing continuous monitoring of blood pressure, you can take frequent blood samples for blood gas analysis without causing further discomfort to the patient.

Using an arterial line

To monitor blood pressure, the arterial line is attached to a transducer. This allows the patient's blood pressure to be displayed as a waveform on a cardiac monitor. The normal set-up for an arterial line is shown in Fig. 2.1 (overpage).

To prevent the backflow of blood along the arterial line and to ensure that the patency of the cannula is maintained, a pressurised normal saline flush of 3 mL/hour is connected to the tubing. The pressure of the flush fluid is maintained at 300 mmHg to ensure it is above arterial pressure (Jevon and Ewens, 2007).

Insertion sites for an arterial line
- Radial artery (*most* common)
- Brachial artery
- Dorsalis pedis
- Femoral artery (*avoid* if possible)

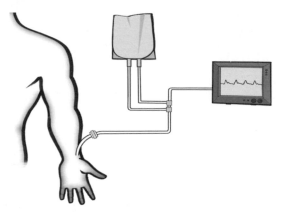

Fig. 2.1 *An arterial line in situ.*

The radial artery

The radial artery is the most commonly used as it is easy to access, reduces patient mobility less than other sites and is easy to monitor and observe. If you do use the radial artery, you should first carry an **Allen's test** to make sure the collateral circulation to the hand is adequate for maintaining perfusion (Haworth *et al.*, 2004).

To carry out the Allen's test, occlude the radial and ulnar arteries until the hand blanches (usually 10 to 30 seconds) then release the pressure on the ulnar artery. Colour should return to the hand within 15 seconds. If it doesn't, you should use an alternative site (Haworth *et al.*, 2004). This is shown in Fig. 2.2.

Complications of an arterial line

- Haemorrhage
- Ischaemia
- Skin and digit necrosis
- Thrombosis
- Air embolism

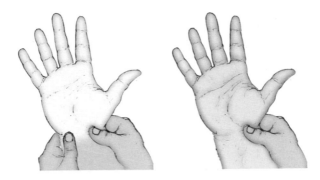

Fig. 2.2 *Allen's test. Left: occlusion of the radial and ulnar arteries and resultant pallor. Right: colour returns to normal on releasing the pressure. From Foxall (2008) with permission from M&K Update.*

The arterial waveform

The arterial waveform seen on the cardiac monitor depicts the pressures within the arteries during the cardiac cycle (Fig. 2.3).

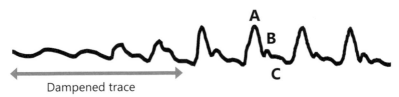

Dampened trace

Fig. 2.3 *The arterial waveform. If the waveform is dampened or flat, check the patient is not in asystole, then manipulate the arm and flush the line to rectify.*

A is the **peak systolic pressure:** this reflects the pressure in the arterial system at the peak of systole.
B is the **dicrotic notch:** this reflects aortic valve closure.
C is the **diastolic pressure:** this reflects the pressure in the arterial system during diastole and therefore the degree of vasoconstriction.
(Adam and Osbourne, 2005)

Arterial line management

Action	Rationale
Always wash your hands thoroughly before handling any part of the system (and handle the system as little as possible)	To prevent infection
The transducer should be calibrated on a regular basis, according to the recommendations of the equipment supplier	To ensure readings are accurate
The transducer should be level with the mid-axillary line (Fig. 2.2) (zero reference point) when calibrating the device and when taking recordings	To ensure readings are accurate
Ensure the flush fluid bag does not run dry and that the pressure bag remains at 300 mmHg (change the flush fluid bag according to local protocol)	To prevent the backflow of blood, clotting within the cannula and possible thrombosis
If the waveform is dampened or flat, check the patient is not in asystole, then manipulate the arm and flush the line to rectify	To ensure readings are accurate and maintain patient safety
Ensure there are no air bubbles in the system	To ensure readings are accurate and prevent air embolism
Use a transparent dressing at the insertion site and ensure the limb is visible at all times (replace the dressing when soiled)	To enable easy monitoring of the site for infection, tissue necrosis and haemorrhage and to maintain patient safety
If the femoral artery has been cannulated, take extra care	The site will not be visible and the fearea is more prone to infection

Action	Rationale
Label the insertion site 'arterial line'	To prevent inadvertent drug administration through the line (this will cause arterial spasm)
Set the monitor alarms to appropriate levels	To maintain patient safety
If the limb is painful, cold, white or blanches when the line is flushed, inform medical staff (the line will need to be removed)	To prevent perfusion problems and to maintain patient safety
If the cannula appears to have clotted, withdraw blood, then flush through NEVER flush a blocked line! ALWAYS withdraw blood before flushing!	To prevent thrombosis and maintain patient safety

Consolidation

See pages 115–116 for answers

2.1   What is the most common means of monitoring blood pressure in the critically ill patient?

_____

2.2   Other than continuous blood pressure monitoring, what use does an indwelling arterial line have?

_____

2.3   Why is it necessary to have a pressurised flush of 3 mL per hour attached to an arterial line?

_____

_____

2.4   Name the main insertion sites for an arterial line.

_____

_____

2.5   Which is the preferred insertion site for an arterial line?

_____

2.6   Why is this so?

_____

_____

2.7   What test is carried out prior to the insertion of a radial arterial line?

_____

2.8   Why is this so?

_____

2.9   Describe this test.

_____

_____

_____

2.10   What are the complications of an arterial line?

_____

_____

2.11   What does the waveform on the cardiac monitor from the arterial line depict?

_____

2.12   What are the points A, B and C on the arterial waveform?

_____

_____

2.13   Explain what these three points represent.

_____

_____

_____

2.14   What actions must be taken to ensure readings remain accurate?

_____

_____

_____

_____

2.15   What actions need to be taken, and why, to maintain patient safety and prevent complications?

_____

_____

_____

_____

_____

Notes

Notes

Chapter 3

Central venous pressure monitoring

Central venous pressure (CVP) reflects right atrial filling pressure as the line sits in the right atrium when in situ (Fig. 3.1). Therefore it may also be referred to as right atrial pressure. A CVP line allows monitoring of venous return and right ventricular function and gives a good indication of fluid status (Jevon and Ewens, 2007).

What is normal CVP?

> **Normal CVP**
> 5–10 cm water *or* 0–8 mmHg

CVP and artificial ventilation

If a patient's CVP is being recorded while he or she is receiving artificial ventilation, the reading will be higher than normal because of increased intrathoracic pressure caused by positive pressure ventilation. In addition, if positive end expiratory pressure (PEEP) is applied, the reading will be even higher and will correlate with the amount of PEEP.

For example:

If the CVP is 16 mmHg and the patient has a PEEP of +6, the reading without PEEP would be 10 mmHg. As the patient is receiving artificial ventilation, you would expect it to be higher than normal. Therefore a CVP of 16 mmHg in this patient is acceptable.

Other uses of CVP lines

In addition to monitoring central venous pressure, central lines have several other uses (Adam and Osborne, 2005). These are:

- to administer large fluid volumes during fluid resuscitation
- to administer parenteral nutrition
- to administer irritant drugs.

The CVP line in situ

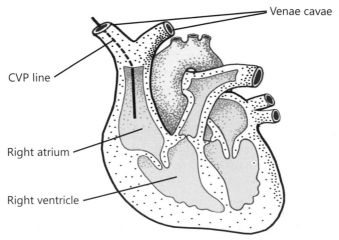

Fig. 3.1 *CVP line in situ.*

Insertion sites for a CVP line

There are three possible sites for insertion, namely:

- The subclavian vein (preferred site).
- The internal jugular vein (least complications).
- The femoral vein (avoid if possible as there is an increased risk of infection because of its position).

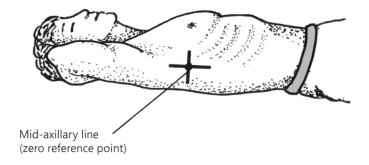

Mid-axillary line
(zero reference point)

Fig. 3.2 *The mid-axillary line.*

Taking CVP measurements

CVP measurements should be taken from a dedicated line to ensure accurate readings are taken.

However, if measurements are to be taken using a central line that is *also* being used as an infusion line, then a falsely high reading may be obtained (Jevon and Ewens, 2007). Infusions should be stopped temporarily to ensure the CVP reading is accurate.

CVP lines are available in single or multilumen versions. Different catheters can be chosen to suit each patient's requirements. The transducer should be level with the mid-axillary line (zero reference point) when calibrating the device and when taking recordings (Fig. 3.2).

To monitor CVP, the CVP line is attached to a transducer. This allows the CVP to be displayed as a waveform on a cardiac monitor.

As with the arterial line, prevent the backflow of blood along the CVP line and ensure patency of the cannula by connecting a pressurised normal saline flush to the tubing set at 3 ml/hour at 300 mmHg.

The CVP waveform

The CVP waveform seen on the cardiac monitor (Fig. 3.3) denotes the pressures within the subclavian veins and right atrium just before the blood enters the right ventricle.

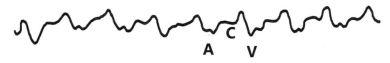

Fig. 3.3 *The CVP waveform.*

Points A, C and V

A represents **right atrial contraction**.
C represents **tricuspid valve closure**.
V represents **ventricular contraction** (which slightly increases right atrial pressure).
(Adam and Osborne, 2005)

What do CVP measurments indicate?

A *low* CVP indicates hypovolaemia and/or vasodilation.
A *high* CVP indicates fluid overload and/or vasoconstriction.

Therefore, CVP monitoring can be very useful in assessing a patient's cardiovascular status. It gives a good indication of:

- Cardiac function
- Vascular tone
- Fluid status.

However, a number of factors can influence CVP readings. This is why a single CVP reading should not be used to titrate intravenous fluids and/or drugs. Trends are far more valuable than single readings.

The CVP should be monitored *as well as* blood pressure and urine output. In this way an overall picture of the patient's condition can be established (Gonce-Morton, 2005).

Complications of a CVP line

Complications of the CVP line include:

- Pneumothorax
- Haemorrhage
- Haematoma
- Infection possibly leading to sepsis
- Air embolism
- Thrombosis
- Cardiac arrhythmias
- Puncture of the vein, atrial or ventricular wall
- Catheter malposition
- Catheter tip embolus

Some of these complications can be avoided by careful management of the CVP line. The specifics of CVP line management are covered in detail in the table overpage.

CVP line management

Action	Rationale
Strict aseptic technique should be observed during insertion. Always wash your hands thoroughly before handling any part of the system (and handle the system as little as possible)	To prevent infection
The transducer should be calibrated on a regular basis, according to the recommendations of the equipment supplier	To ensure readings are accurate
The transducer should be level with the mid-axillary line (Fig. 3.2) (zero reference point) when calibrating the device and when taking recordings	To ensure readings are accurate
Ensure the flush fluid bag does not run dry and that the pressure bag remains at 300 mmHg (change the flush fluid bag according to local protocol)	To prevent the backflow of blood, clotting within the cannula and possible thrombosis
Ensure there are no air bubbles in the system	To ensure readings are accurate and prevent air embolism
Use a transparent dressing at the insertion site and ensure the limb is visible at all times Replace the dressing when soiled If the femoral artery has been cannulated, take extra care	To enable easy monitoring of the site for infection, tissue necrosis and haemorrhage and to maintain patient safety The site will not be visible and the area is more prone to infection

Action	Rationale
Set the monitor alarms to appropriate levels	To maintain patient safety
If the cannula appears to have clotted, there will be a high reading with a dampened or flat trace. Ensure patency by withdrawing blood, then flush through NEVER flush a blocked line! ALWAYS withdraw blood before flushing!	To ensure readings are accurate, to prevent thrombosis and to maintain patient safety
If the CVP is unexpectedly high, it is likely the catheter tip is in the right ventricle, which should be confirmed by x-ray (and the catheter should be repositioned by medical staff)	To ensure readings are accurate and maintain patient safety

Consolidation

See page 117 for answers

3.1   What does CVP reflect?

_____

3.2   What is the normal CVP?

_____

3.3   What effect does artificial ventilation have on CVP?

_____

_____

3.4   What effect does PEEP have on CVP?

_____

_____

3.5   In addition to monitoring CVP, what are central lines used for?

_____

_____

3.6   What are the insertion sites for CVP lines?

_____

3.7   Why is it best to avoid the femoral vein?

_____

3.8   What do the points A, C and V on the CVP waveform denote?

_____

_____

_____

3.9   What does a low CVP indicate?

_____

3.10   What does a high CVP indicate?

_____

3.11   What other variables should be monitored in conjunction with CVP?

_____

_____

3.12   Why is this so?

_____

_____

3.13   What are the complications of a CVP line?

_____

_____

_____

3.14   What are the nursing considerations for a patient with a CVP line in situ for ensuring safety is maintained?

_____

_____

_____

_____

_____

3.15   If there is a high reading with a dampened or flat trace, what action would you take?

_____

_____

3.16   If the CVP is unexpectedly high, what action would you take?

_____

_____

Notes

Notes

Chapter 4

Monitoring and maintenance of cardiac output and tissue perfusion

Accurate clinical assessment is particularly important in critically ill patients, whose haemodynamic status may change rapidly. Continuous monitoring of cardiac output will provide information that allows rapid adjustment of therapy (Jansen, 2002). The pulmonary artery catheter is useful for evaluating the function of the heart and can detect developing problems in the vasculature of the lungs. Optimisation of oxygen delivery to the tissues is facilitated by the titration of drugs that affect cardiac output and peripheral resistance.

The pulmonary artery catheter

The pulmonary artery catheter (PAC) was first introduced in 1970 by Swan and Ganz (hence it is often known as a Swan–Ganz catheter. It has been generally accepted as the 'gold standard' against which all other methods of cardiac output monitoring are compared (Jansen, 2002; Pybus *et al.*, 2000).

Many new methods have been used in an attempt to replace the PAC, mainly because it is so invasive. The principles of cardiac output measurement are the same whichever system is used, but non-PAC methods do not measure all the parameters that a PAC does.

Cardiac output monitoring

For the purpose of this workbook, we are going to describe the use of the PAC in detail, but the principles and management of the PAC also apply to other monitoring techniques. Alternative monitoring techniques are:

1. Transoesophageal echo-Doppler ultrasound

The oesophageal Doppler technique measures blood flow velocity in the aorta and hence cardiac output. The Doppler transducer is in the tip of a flexible probe which is sited in the patient's oesophagus (Berton and Cholley, 2002).

2. Methods employing the Fick principle

An example of this is the NICO system (Novametrix). This non-invasive device uses the Fick principle to measure the difference between the arterial level and the venous level of carbon dioxide (arterial CO_2 *minus* venous CO_2). In accordance with the Fick principle, cardiac output can be calculated from the ratio of oxygen consumption and the difference in oxygen levels between the arteries and veins (as with carbon dioxide) (Berton and Cholley, 2002).

3. Arterial pulse contour analysis

Examples of these are the PiCCO (Pulsion) and the PulseCO (LiDCO) systems. The technique involves measuring and monitoring stroke volume on a beat-by-beat basis from the arterial pulse pressure waveform (via an arterial line). Cardiac output can then be calculated by relating an arterial pressure or pressure difference to a flow or volume change (Pinskey and Payne, 2005).

The lumens of a PAC

PACs are available with up to six lumens (Haworth *et al.*, 2004), but the five-lumen PAC (Fig. 4.1) is the most commonly used.

(1) The **balloon port lumen** is used to inflate and deflate the thin latex

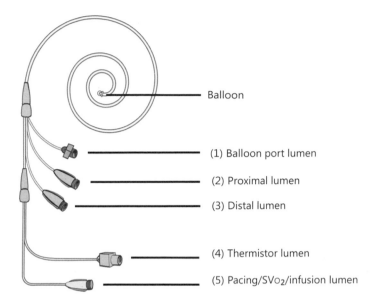

Fig. 4.1 *The components of a five-lumen PAC. The balloon port lumen (1) always has a Luer-locked syringe attached.*

balloon that surrounds – but does not cover – the tip of the catheter when inflated and measures pulmonary artery wedge pressure (PAWP).

(2) The **proximal lumen** measures CVP (the opening is 30 cm from the tip).

(3) The **distal lumen** measures pulmonary artery pressure (PAP) (the opening is located at the tip).

(4) The **thermistor lumen** contains a temperature-sensitive wire for determining cardiac output by thermodilution.

(5) **Additional lumens** are used for infusing fluids and/or drugs or they may provide a port for pacemaker electrodes or continuous measurement of mixed venous oxygen saturation (Haworth *et al.*, 2004).

Insertion of the PAC

The PAC is inserted via the venous system through the right heart and into the pulmonary circulation, assisted by balloon flotation (Fig. 4.2). It enables pressures to be monitored throughout the heart and cardiovascular system and allows cardiac output to be measured by thermodilution (Pybus *et al.*, 2000).

The PAC is inserted into the superior vena cava, usually via the subclavian or jugular vein. From the vena cava it passes into the right atrium. The balloon is then inflated and floats into the right ventricle through the tricuspid valve, then through the pulmonary valve into a branch of the pulmonary artery. It wedges here when the balloon is inflated. The full name for this device is the multi-lumen, thermodilution, pulmonary artery flotation catheter.

The PAC is important for monitoring the patient's haemodynamic status. It guides therapy relating to fluid balance and aids in the implementation and evaluation of appropriate pharmacological support.

Indications for insertion of a PAC

The cardiovascular system is a continuous loop system driven by the heart. However, there are pressure gradients throughout the system that ensure the blood keeps moving around the body. Any condition that affects the circulation requires monitoring. Clearly, the more severe the condition, the more closely it needs to be monitored. The insertion of a PAC is indicated when there is impaired cardiac function and/or pulmonary hypertension. It ensures that fluid management optimises circulatory volume and/or that inotropic or vasoactive agents optimise oxygen delivery.

Complications of a PAC

The PAC is a very invasive monitoring technique so there are a few complications to look out for. If there is any sign of any of the complications listed below, inform a senior member of staff immediately.

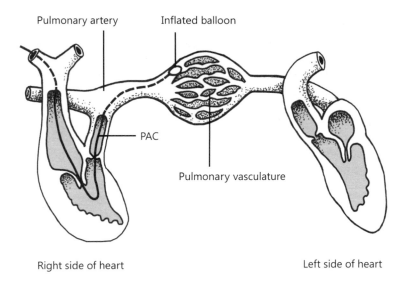

Fig. 4.2 *Expanded view of the PAC in situ.*

Complications on insertion

- Ventricular arrhythmias
- Pneumothorax
- Arterial puncture
- Air embolism (may be caused by balloon rupture)
- Myocardial perforation

Longer term complications

- Kinking of the tube (leads to blockage)
- Sepsis
- Thrombosis
- Catheter embolus
- Pulmonary infarction (caused by spontaneous or over-wedging)

Pressure waveforms

As the PAC passes through the heart, the waveform changes. (You should also observe for arrhythmias.)

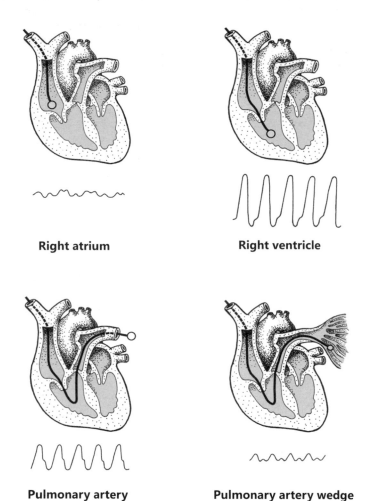

Right atrium

Right ventricle

Pulmonary artery

Pulmonary artery wedge

Fig. 4.3 *Normal PAC waveforms.*

Nursing responsibilities during insertion of the PAC

Action	Rationale
Prepare all necessary equipment, ensuring asepsis	To ensure all equipment is ready and close to hand and to prevent infection
Make sure (as far as possible) that the patient is fully aware of what is going to happen	To gain consent and cooperation
Position the patient on his or her back with the foot of the bed raised	To engorge the neck veins to make them easier to locate and to prevent air embolism
Observe the pressure traces as the PAC passes through the chambers of the heart	To ensure the PAC is being positioned correctly
Observe the cardiac monitor for arrhythmias	To ensure swift resolution of problems
Monitor vital signs	To ensure swift resolution of problems
Assist the doctor	To ensure a smooth procedure
Give explanations and reassurance to the patient throughout the procedure	To reduce anxiety

N.B. Always follow local policy and procedure when assisting with insertion of a PAC, zero referencing and calibrating equipment. If you are unsure of anything, ask a senior member of staff.

Nursing responsibilities when a PAC is in situ

Action	Rationale
Zero reference and calibrate equipment when taking over the care of the patient	To ensure readings are accurate
Always ensure the pulmonary artery pressure (PAP) trace is visible on the monitor (see Fig. 4.4)	To monitor for spontaneous wedging and therefore maintain patient safety
Observe the insertion site for infection or bleeding	To ensure any problems are dealt with swiftly
Make sure the catheter does not kink	To prevent blockage of the line and ensure readings are accurate
Ensure correct flushing	To prevent blockage of the line

Parameters measured by the PAC

Central venous pressure (CVP)

This was discussed in Chapter 3.

Pulmonary artery pressure (PAP)

See Fig. 4.4. PAP reflects **right ventricular pressure**. It also indicates resistance in the pulmonary vascular bed due to reduced pulmonary blood flow, usually because of pulmonary hypertension or regurgitation of blood. Therefore, if the PAP is raised, there is congestion of blood in the lungs. This can mean there is a problem on the left side of the heart because it is not ejecting the stroke volume adequately, leading to back-pressure.

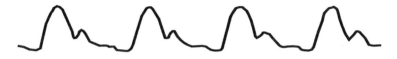

Pulmonary artery pressure (PAP)

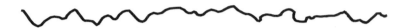

Pulmonary artery wedge pressure (PAWP)

Fig. 4.4 *PAP (upper trace) and PAWP (lower trace) waveforms.*

Pulmonary artery wedge pressure (PAWP)

You may also hear PAWP being referred to as **pulmonary capillary wedge pressure** (PCWP), **pulmonary artery occlusion pressure** (PAOP) or simply **wedge pressure**.

PAWP indicates **preload**, which is the pressure in the left ventricle at the end of diastole. Therefore, left ventricular end-diastolic pressure equals PAWP, thus:

$$LVEDP = PAWP$$

If PAP is raised, PAWP is *also* raised because both are affected by congestion of blood in the lungs (which increases pressure). PAWP correlates with PAP diastolic pressure (Jevon and Ewens, 2007) (see Fig. 4.5).

Normal PAP and PAWP

PAP 20–30 mmHg (systolic) *or* 10–20 mmHg (diastolic)

PAWP 8–15 mmHg

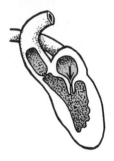

Left ventricle fills with blood.

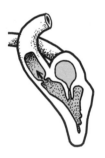

Left ventricle cannot contract forcefully enough to completely eject the stroke volume.

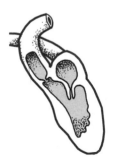

Ventricle should be empty but some blood remains.

Figure 4.5 *Pressure increase in the left ventricle.*

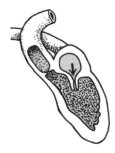

Left atrium empties blood into the ventricle as some of the last stroke volume remains, blood volume increases, increasing end diastolic pressure.

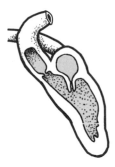

Left ventricle contracts, but not with enough force to eject the even larger stroke volume.

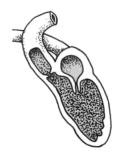

Stroke volume increases, as does end-diastolic pressure, and blood flow becomes more sluggish (like a traffic jam). As a result, pressure within the pulmonary vasculature starts to increase, demonstrated by increased PAP and PAWP. This continues, worsening the patient's condition. Drug therapy is required to increase cardiac contractility to clear the backlog of blood and increase blood flow.

Procedure for undertaking PAWP measurements

Action	Rationale
1. Wash your hands	To maintain a clean environment and prevent infection
2. Inform the patient of your actions	To obtain consent and cooperation
3. Slowly inflate the balloon with no more than 1.5 mL of air. Continue to watch the monitor until the flattened wedge waveform is visible (see Fig. 4.3)	To avoid over-inflation of the balloon (could cause vessel damage or balloon rupture). The balloon is now 'wedged' in a branch of the pulmonary artery
4. Allow the trace to run for three respiratory cycles (approximately 15 seconds)	To provide an accurate reading while avoiding pulmonary infarction
5. Freeze the monitor screen and deflate the balloon	To provide an accurate reading while avoiding pulmonary infarction
6. Record the wedge pressure according to equipment instructions	To ensure an accurate reading
7. Unfreeze the screen and ensure the PAP trace is present	To maintain patient safety

N.B. This is a generic procedure that may detract from local policy, and is for guidance only, Always follow your local policy. Only trained staff should carry out the procedure. Some monitors capture data automatically. Always follow the instructions provided by the equipment supplier.

Once the results are available, ensure they are appropriately documented and inform medical staff if necessary.

Cardiac output (CO)

> **Normal CO**
> Approximately 5 litres per minute

Cardiac output (CO) is the amount of blood ejected from the left ventricle in 1 minute.

It is calculated by multiplying the stroke volume by the heart rate. The **stroke volume** is the amount of blood ejected from the left ventricle during each heartbeat and it is normally 70 mL. Normal **heart rate** is approximately 72 beats per minute (b.p.m.). Therefore,

CO = stroke volume (70 mL) × heart rate (72 b.p.m.)
CO = 70 × 72
CO = 5040 mL (i.e. approximately 5 litre/min)

A **low cardiac output** indicates inefficient pumping action of the heart (pump failure), such as that seen in cardiogenic shock or the final stage of septic shock (more about this in Chapter 5).

A **high cardiac output** indicates a hyperdynamic state, such as that seen in the warm shock phase of septic shock (more about this in Chapter 5).

Thermodilution

A bolus of fluid, usually 10 mL of 5% dextrose, is rapidly injected (within 4 seconds) into the right atrium through the proximal port of the PAC. This is done at least three times and an average is then calculated. The injection fluid must be cooler than the patient's blood to bring about a temperature change which can be sensed by the thermistor. The temperature change that occurs as the bolus mixes with the stroke volume pumped out of the right ventricle is 'read' downstream by the thermistor in the pulmonary artery. The signal is then transmitted back through the thermistor wires to the cardiac monitor and displayed in litres per minute.

Cardiac index (CI)

> **Normal CI**
> 2.8–3.6 litres per min/m²

As we have seen, cardiac output is approximately 5 litres per minute, but not all patients are the same size! Obviously output measurements will differ between different patients, so the **cardiac index** gives an individual body-size-related measurement, calculated from height and weight, which allows us to compare cardiac output values in different patients (Fig. 4.6).

What is the effect of body size on cardiac output?

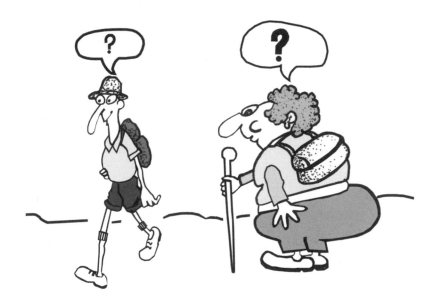

Fig. 4.6 *Patients can have very different body sizes. In order to compare cardiac output values, differences in their sizes can be minimised by calculating cardiac index.*

Cardiac index is calculated by dividing the cardiac output by body surface area in square metres:

$$CI = \text{cardiac output (L/min)} \div \text{body surface area (m}^2)$$

A **low cardiac index** (like low cardiac output) indicates inefficient pump action of the heart (**pump failure**) and may be seen in cardiogenic shock or the final stage of septic shock (covered in Chapter 5).

A **high cardiac index** (like high cardiac output) indicates a hyperdynamic state like that seen in the warm shock phase of septic shock (this is also covered in Chapter 5).

Cardiac output and cardiac index will *always* correlate. This means, if one rises, the other will too.

Systemic vascular resistance (SVR)

> **Normal SVR**
> 700–1200 dynes

Systemic vascular resistance (SVR) indicates **afterload**, which is the amount of resistance that the ventricle has to overcome in order to eject the stroke volume. In a hose-pipe, the narrower the tube, the higher the pressure.

Similarly, if the circulation is vasoconstricted, the heart has to work harder to work to maintain the circulation. If there is vasodilation, there is less pressure for the heart to work against.

A **low SVR** (below 700) indicates **vasodilation**, like that seen in the warm shock phase of sepsis (see Chapter 5).

A **high SVR** (more than 1200) indicates **vasoconstriction**, which is the response of the sympathetic nervous system to low cardiac output and therefore low blood pressure.

Indexed systemic vascular resistance (SVRi)

Like cardiac index, SVR can be *indexed* to body surface area. This is denoted by the term SVRi.

> **Normal SVRi**
> 900–1400

Mixed venous oxygen saturation (SVO$_2$)

> **Normal SVO$_2$**
> 75%
> (% of oxygenated blood returning to the heart)

Mixed venous oxygen saturation (SVO$_2$) refers to the amount of oxygen that remains in the blood at the end of the circulation (after tissue perfusion). It is dependent on the haemoglobin content of the blood, oxygen saturation and cardiac output. It reflects the body's ability to supply enough oxygen to meet the metabolic demands of the tissues (Viney, 1999). It also gives an indication of the difference between oxygen delivery and oxygen consumption (Pybus *et al.*, 2000).

A **low SVO$_2$** indicates that oxygen delivery is reduced, tissue oxygen demand is increased, or both (i.e. there is an imbalance between oxygen supply and demand). SVO$_2$ needs to be higher than 30% to meet the minimum oxygen requirements of the tissues (Jevon and Ewens, 2007).

A **high SVO$_2$** indicates that oxygen uptake by the tissues is reduced. The most common cause of a high SVO$_2$ is sepsis when there is a hyperdynamic circulation. This is because oxygen is available within the circulation but is not taken up appropriately by the tissues (see Chapter 5).

N.B. There are other parameters that are measured by the PAC but the ones outlined above are considered the most important and reflect the pressures throughout the heart and cardiovascular system.

Consolidation

See pages 118–121 for answers

4.1   Name four ways of measuring cardiac output.

4.2   What is a pulmonary artery catheter?

4.3   Name the lumens in a PAC and describe what each is used for.

4.4   What would you do, and why, to prepare a patient for the insertion of a PAC?

4.5   What are the responsibilities of the nurse assisting the doctor during insertion of a PAC?

_____

_____

_____

_____

4.6   What are the nursing responsibilities for patients with a PAC in situ?

_____

_____

_____

_____

4.7   What are the complications of a PAC?

_____

_____

_____

4.8   Which parameters does a PAC measure?

_____

_____

_____

_____

4.9   What does PAP stand for?

4.10   What is the normal PAP?

4.11   What does PAP indicate?

4.12   What does a raised PAP indicate?

4.13   What does PAWP stand for?

4.14   What is the normal PAWP?

4.15   What does PAWP indicate?

4.16   Explain the term preload.

4.17   With which other parameter does PAWP correlate?

4.18   What does a raised PAWP indicate?

_____

_____

4.19   How is PAWP measured?

_____

_____

_____

_____

4.20   What is the maximum amount of air that should be used to inflate the balloon to measure PAWP?

_____

4.21   Where does the balloon wedge?

_____

4.22   Which waveform should be constantly displayed on the cardiac monitor when a PAC is in situ?

_____

4.23   Why is this so?

_____

4.24   What is the cardiac output and what is its normal value?

_____

_____

If, in your clinical area, you are able to undertake PAWP measurements, under the supervision of your mentor, take five measurements, following local procedure. Discuss any issues with your mentor. Record your progress in the following table.

	Date	Comments	Signature of mentor
Measurement 1			
Measurement 2			
Measurement 3			
Measurement 4			
Measurement 5			

4.25   How is cardiac output calculated?

_____

4.26   What does a low cardiac output indicate?

_____

_____

4.27   What does a high cardiac output indicate?

_____

_____

4.28   What is the cardiac index and what is its normal value?

_____

_____

4.29   What is the significance of the cardiac index?

_____

_____

4.30   How is cardiac index calculated?

_____

_____

4.31   What does a low cardiac index indicate?

_____

_____

4.32   What does a high cardiac index indicate?

_____

_____

4.33   How is cardiac output measured using a PAC?

_____

_____

_____

_____

4.34   How many times should this be carried out so that an average cardiac output can be calculated?

_____

4.35   Why must the injection fluid be cooler than the patient's blood?

_____

4.36   What does SVR stand for?

_____

4.37   What is the normal SVR?

_____

4.38   What does SVR indicate?

_____

_____

4.39   What does a high SVR indicate?

_____

4.40   What does a low SVR indicate?

_____

4.41   What does SVRi stand for?

_____

4.42   What is the normal SVRi?

_____

4.43   Explain the term 'mixed venous oxygen saturation' (SVO_2).

_____

_____

4.44   What is the normal SVO_2?

_____

4.45   What does a low SVO_2 indicate?

_____

_____

4.46   What does a high SVO_2 indicate?

_____

_____

4.47   What does an SVO_2 of less than 30% indicate?

_____

_____

Notes

Notes

Chapter 5

The effects of shock

Shock is a syndrome which results in inadequate tissue perfusion and is classified according to its aetiology.

Definition of shock

Shock can be defined as acute circulatory failure with inadequate or inappropriately distributed tissue perfusion resulting in generalised cellular hypoxia (Graham and Parke, 2005). Or, more simply, it is **inadequate tissue perfusion due to reduced blood flow**.

What happens in shock?

If blood flow is reduced the tissues will not receive sufficient oxygen or nutrients and waste products will not be removed – leading to cellular hypoxia and starvation, then cell death, organ dysfunction, organ failure, and eventually death (Hand, 2001). Let's look at this in more detail. Reduced tissue perfusion:

- leads to a reduction in venous return, and therefore cardiac output, which will lead to low blood pressure – which further reduces tissue perfusion
- stimulates the sympathetic nervous system to release catecholamines, adrenaline and noradrenaline, that cause peripheral vasoconstriction – and further reduces tissue perfusion
- instigates anaerobic respiration due to hypoxia and the end-product of hypoxia is lactic acid; therefore acidosis develops and this leads to myocardial failure.

Catecholamines also cause tachycardia and increased myocardial contractility which increases myocardial oxygen demand while the supply is reduced, leading to myocardial failure. This in turn causes multiple organ failure, leading to multi-organ dysfunction syndrome (MODS) and ultimately death. See Fig. 5.1.

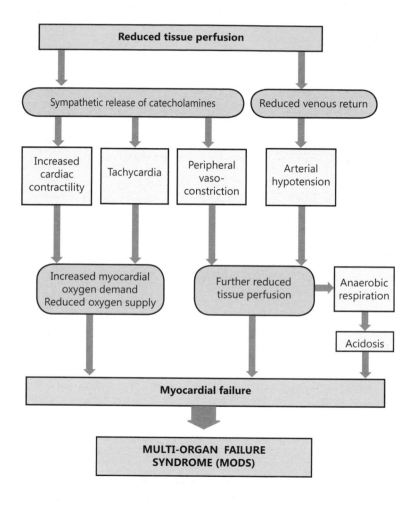

Fig. 5.1 *The effects of shock.*

Shock is generally easily to recognise from basic clinical signs such as heart rate, blood pressure, colour, capillary refill time and alterations in mental status (lethargy, confusion or deterioration in conscious level). However, haemodynamic monitoring enables medical and nursing staff to differentiate between the different shock states. Therefore it helps them to diagnose the type and level of shock, to manage symptoms by titration of drugs and fluids and to evaluate the treatments instigated (Pybus *et al.*, 2000).

Stages of shock

There are four stages of shock, relating to the severity of the physiological response. Each stage has distinct clinical characteristics (Table 5.1).

Table 5.1 The clinical characteristics of the stages of shock

	Physiological response	**Physiological effects**
STAGE 1 Early shock	Increased sympathetic discharge	Normal blood pressure Tachycardia Rapid breathing Diaphoresis (sweating) Dilated pupils Anxiety
STAGE 2 Middle shock	Decreased organ perfusion	Blood pressure reducing (may be normal) Tachycardia Lethargy Disorientation Decreased urine output Cool clammy skin
STAGE 3 Late shock	Failure of compensatory mechanisms	Hypotension Weak thready pulse Altered conscious state Anuria Skin cold to the touch
STAGE 4 Fourth-stage shock	Multiple organ dysfunction syndrome (MODS)	Loss of function in major organs (lungs, kidneys, liver) Severe cardiovascular instability Loss of host defences Coagulopathy

Principles of shock management

Regardless of the type or stage of shock, the principles of shock management are the same, that is **to maintain adequate oxygen delivery to the tissues**.

1. Provide respiratory support

Depending on the patient's respiratory status, measures will range from oxygen administration to artificial ventilation. There must be adequate oxygen intake to supply tissue oxygen demand.

2. Maintain and/or improve circulating volume

This may be in the form of intravenous fluids or blood products, depending on the nature of the shock state.

3. Improve cardiac output and/or vascular tone

If oxygen intake is adequate and there is sufficient fluid or blood in the circulation to carry oxygen, the heart still needs to be able to pump effectively to ensure adequate oxygen delivery. In certain shock states, this may require inotropic agents that increase cardiac contractility and therefore cardiac output; in other shock states, vasodilation reduces blood pressure so vasoactive agents are required to constrict the circulation to increase blood pressure. Many times, both types of drug are required (see Chapter 6).

4. Maintain renal function

The blood pressure needs to be maintained to ensure there is sufficient pressure to filter blood in the glomerulus of the kidney. If the heart is pumping ineffectively, renal blood flow is affected and urine output reduces. If this is not swiftly rectified, acute renal failure follows.

5. Eradicate any source of infection

Systemic infection will lead to sepsis and septic shock. Where this is suspected, early diagnosis and treatment is essential.

Types of shock

Shock is divided into four categories:

- hypovolaemic shock
- obstructive shock
- cardiogenic shock
- distributive shock.

1. Hypovolaemic shock

Hypovolaemic shock results from loss of circulating volume even if the heart is pumping adequately. Reduced circulating volume is caused by external fluid loss or internal fluid shifts, hence inadequate tissue perfusion (Diehl-Oplinger and Kaminski, 2004). A reduced oxygen supply to the heart eventually results in cardiovascular failure, worsening the shock state. Causes include:

- external haemorrhage
- internal haemorrhage (e.g. gastrointestinal bleeding)
- fractures
- major fluid loss (e.g. vomiting, diarrhoea, sweating)
- renal failure
- excessive diuretic use
- burns
- sepsis.

2. Obstructive shock

Obstructive shock, as you might expect, is caused by an obstruction in the circulation. This obstruction means venous return is reduced, and therefore so is cardiac output. Vasoconstriction occurs in an attempt to maintain blood pressure as a result of the compensatory action of the sympathetic nervous system. Causes include:

- tension pneumothorax
- cardiac tamponade
- pulmonary embolism
- aortic aneurysm
- aortic stenosis.

Septic shock

The aetiology of septic shock is not as yet fully understood but because it is the most commonly occurring type of shock in critical and acute care we will discuss it in detail. You may also know it as:

- **gram-negative sepsis** because it is often (but not always) caused by gram-negative bacteria, or
- **endotoxic shock** because it occurs as a result of the body's immune and inflammatory responses to the endotoxins released when the cell wall of bacteria is destroyed (Chamberlain, 2004).

It spreads most commonly through poor hand washing, and it is considered to be a very dangerous nosocomial (hospital-acquired) infection, with increasing incidence and a high mortality rate (Filbin and Stapczynski, 2006). Usually it occurs in a vulnerable host (that is, someone whose health is already compromised), caused by an aggressive guest, often a normally symbiotic resident of the gut such as *Escherichia coli*, *Klebsiella* or *Pseudomonas* (Filbin and Stapczynski, 2006). The inflammatory response leads to increased permeability of the blood vessels, which allows bacteria to get into the blood. Rapid systemic infection follows (Sharma, 2007).

The stages of septic shock

1. Systemic inflammatory response syndrome (SIRS)
2. Sepsis
3. Severe sepsis
4. Septic shock

Stage 1: Systemic inflammatory response syndrome (SIRS)

Body temperature alters (usually above 38°C, but sometimes below 36°C). Heart rate increases to over 90 b.p.m. Respiratory rate increases to over 20 breaths per minute, causing a decrease in blood carbon dioxide levels (PCO_2) of less than 4.0 kPa and therefore a respiratory alkalosis (Chamberlain, 2004). In addition, the white blood cell count rises as more cells are produced to fight the infection (Sharma, 2007).

Stage 2: Sepsis

Sepsis occurs when SIRS is present and blood culture results are positive.

Stage 3: Severe sepsis

Severe sepsis occurs when sepsis is present and there is also organ dysfunction with hypotension and/or hypoperfusion abnormalities (may manifest as hypoxia, lactic acidosis, oliguria or acute alteration in mental status, or a combination of these).

Stage 4: Septic shock

Septic shock occurs when severe sepsis is present with hypoperfusion abnormalities and hypotension that does not respond to fluid resuscitation. There are *two types* of septic shock, namely:

- **warm** shock (also known as hyperdynamic shock) and
- **cold** shock (also known as hypodynamic shock).

We will describe both in some detail.

The warm phase of septic shock

This occurs first. It is characterised by high cardiac output, low systemic vascular resistance (SVR) and low blood pressure as vasodilation occurs from the effects of histamine, serotonin and endorphins released during the inflammatory response. Capillaries also become more permeable, causing leakage of fluid into the tissues and leading to a relative hypovolaemia. Several other factors lead to further fluid loss:

- **Fever** (leads to diaphoresis; it is caused by a substance known as endogenous pyrogen which is released by leucocytes when attacking gram-negative bacteria).
- **Increased respiratory rate** (leads to further loss of water vapour).
- **Profound diuresis** (results from a high osmotic load, caused by breakdown of dead bacteria and tissue).

Coagulopathy (abnormal clotting) occurs, with the formation of multiple fibrin clots that obstruct small capillaries. This manifests as a 'creeping' mottling of the legs. **Disseminated intravascular coagulation** (DIC) is often a complication (Filbin and Stapczynski, 2006).

In warm shock, oxygen uptake and delivery is impaired and therefore anaerobic respiration occurs (causing a metabolic acidosis, as lactic acid is the end-product of anaerobic respiration). The acidosis will be seen as a base deficit. Blood oxygen concentration (PO_2) may be elevated in the early stages because of the high respiratory rate and (PCO_2) may be profoundly low, also as a result of the high respiratory rate. Respiratory alkalosis will follow, which may counterbalance the lactic acidosis and shift the pH towards alkalosis. The management of warm shock is described in Table 5.2; the haemodynamic changes are shown in Table 5.3 (overpage).

A patient in warm shock will be seriously ill and may deteriorate rapidly, so swift and appropriate treatment must be instigated to prevent worsening of the patient's condition. Activated protein C (Xigris) is now often used in septic patients because it mediates many actions of homeostasis. It is a potent suppressant of inflammation, and it prevents microcoagulation and reverses impaired fibrinolysis (Chamberlain, 2004).

Table 5.2 The management of warm shock

Action	Rationale
Artificial ventilation	To ensure appropriate oxygen delivery
Fluid load (cautiously)	To optimise fluid volume (due to risk of myocardial depression and heart failure)
Fresh frozen plasma	To increase clotting factors and prevent coagulopathy
Antibiotics (give cautiously)	To eradicate the infection (the circulation must be stabilised first or the antibiotics will cause further bacterial destruction and release of endotoxins)
Reduce temperature (if hyperpyrexia present)	To avoid central nervous system damage
Vasopressor e.g. norepinephrine (α1 receptor stimulator) to constrict circulation (see Chapter 6)	To support the cardiovascular system once the circulation is loaded
Inotrope e.g. dobutamine (β1 receptor stimulator) to increase cardiac contractility (see Chapter 6)	To support the cardiovascular system once the circulation is loaded
Calcium (may be given)	To support the cardiovascular system

If warm shock is left untreated or if the infection and symptoms are overwhelming, treatment is rendered ineffective and cold shock occurs.

The cold phase of septic shock

In cold shock, the cardiovascular system fails due to the increased oxygen demand of the hyperdynamic circulation which is failing to supply sufficient oxygen.

Symptoms of cold shock

- Reduced cerebral perfusion (signs of impaired mental status)
- Subnormal temperature
- Low white blood cell count (with many immature cells)
- Profound hypotension and hypoperfusion
- Cold and mottled skin
- Increased heart rate and respirations (because of increased catecholamine levels)
- Reduced cardiac output (due to myocardial depressant factor, released because of vasoconstriction and coagulopathy)

Ultimately, cold shock leads to multiple organ dysfunction syndrome (MODS) resulting in pulmonary oedema, acute respiratory distress syndrome (ARDS), cardiovascular failure, liver and kidney failure, disseminated intravascular coagulation, haemorrhaging and altered consciousness.

Arterial blood gases will demonstrate uncompensated hypoxia and acidosis (Pybus *et al.*, 2000). All supportive measures are given to support the cardiovascular system as far as possible.

The haemodynamic changes occuring in the cold phase of septic shock are shown in Table 5.3 overpage.

Haemodynamic changes in cardiogenic and septic shock

Table 5.3 Effects of cardiogenic and septic shock on haemodynamic parameters and actions required to restore physiological function

Parameter	Cardiogenic shock (pump failure)	Septic shock warm phase	Septic shock cold phase
HR	↑	↑	↓
BP	↓	↓	↓
PAP	↑	↓	↑
PAWP	↑	↓	↑
CVP	↑	↓	↑
CO	↓	↑	↓
CI	↓	↑	↓
SVR	↑	↓	↑
SVo$_2$	↓	↑	↓
Physiological effects	Inadequate pump Preload and afterload are high (i.e. pulmonary congestion and vasoconstriction lead to poor oxygen delivery)	Hyperdynamic circulation (i.e. high cardiac output with low systemic vascular resistance due to vasodilation leading to poor oxygen delivery)	Preload and afterload are high (i.e. pulmonary congestion and vasoconstriction, leading to poor oxygen delivery) Blood pressure is low as the heart is not pumping effectively
Action required	Vasodilate to reduce afterload (with caution so BP does not fall further) Increase cardiac contractility to clear congestion (so reducing preload)	Fluid load Increase cardiac contractility, preload and afterload using an inotrope and vasoconstrictor	Vasodilate to reduce afterload (with caution so BP does not fall further) Increase cardiac contractility to clear congestion (so reducing preload)

Consolidation

See pages 122–124 for answers

5.1 Define shock.

5.2 What are the effects of reduced blood flow?

5.3 Briefly describe the physiological effects of shock.

5.4 What are the four *stages* of shock?

5.5   What is the physiological response to early shock?

_____

5.6   What physiological effects does this response have?

_____

_____

5.7   What is the physiological response to middle shock?

_____

5.8   What physiological effects does this response have?

_____

_____

5.9   What is the physiological response to late shock?

_____

5.10   What physiological effects does this response have?

_____

_____

5.11   What is the physiological response to fourth-stage shock?

_____

5.12   What physiological effects does this response have?

_____

_____

5.13   What are the five principles of shock management?

_____

_____

_____

_____

_____

5.14   What are the four *types* of shock?

_____

5.15   Briefly describe hypovolaemic shock.

_____

_____

_____

5.16   What are the causes of hypovolaemic shock?

_____

_____

5.17   Briefly describe obstructive shock.

_____

_____

5.18   What are the causes of obstructive shock?

_____

_____

5.19   Briefly describe cardiogenic shock.

_____

_____

_____

5.20   What are the causes of cardiogenic shock?

_____

_____

5.21   Briefly describe distributive shock.

_____

_____

_____

5.22   What are the causes of distributive shock?

_____

_____

_____

5.23   What is the most common type of distributive shock seen in critical care units?

_____

5.24   What other two names are given to septic shock and why?

_____

_____

5.25   Which bacteria most commonly cause septic shock?

_____

5.26   How does septic shock occur?

_____

_____

5.27   Name the four stages of the septic process.

_____

_____

5.28   What are the symptoms of SIRS?

_____

_____

_____

_____

5.29   How is sepsis recognised?

_____

5.30   How is severe sepsis recognised?

_____

5.31   How is septic shock recognised?

_____

5.32   Name the two types of septic shock.

_____

_____

5.33   How is warm shock characterised?

_____

_____

5.34   What other factors lead to fluid loss during warm shock?

_____

_____

_____

_____

_____

5.35   How does coagulopathy manifest?

_____

_____

5.36   Complete the table below with arrows for increased and decreased values as appropriate.

Parameter	Cardiogenic shock (pump failure)	Septic shock warm phase	Septic shock cold phase
HR			
BP			
PAP			
PAWP			
CVP			
CO			
CI			
SVR			
SVO$_2$			
Physiological effect			

Notes

Chapter 6

Use and effects of inotropic and vasoactive agents

In the critically ill patient it is of paramount importance to maintain adequate tissue perfusion, and therefore oxygen delivery, to meet the patient's cellular metabolic requirements. These metabolic requirements increase with the stress of the disease processes (Filbin and Stapczynski, 2006).

Oxygen delivery

Oxygen delivery to the cell is dependent on the *oxygen content* of the blood and *cardiac output*.

- Oxygen content varies with the amount of haemoglobin present in the blood and the degree of arterial oxygen saturation.
- Cardiac output depends on preload, myocardial contractility and afterload.

Inotropes and vasoactive drugs can be manipulated to support the patient haemodynamically and hence maintain tissue perfusion (Chamberlain, 2004). Critically ill patients often require inotropic support and/or the use of vasoactive drugs to stabilise their circulation, by maintaining or increasing cardiac output and/or improving vascular tone, which will optimise blood flow and thus oxygen delivery.

However, such drugs will not have this effect unless the cardiorespiratory system is in an appropriate state to render them efficient. Three factors have to be considered and acted upon where necessary, either before or in conjunction with drug therapy (Lisbon, 2003).

These three factors are:

- Fluid load (to optimise cardiac filling pressures).
- Blood products (if necessary, to increase haemoglobin).
- Oxygen inhalation and/or mechanical ventilation (to ensure there is sufficient oxygen in the blood).

Inotropy is the regulation of the force of myocardial contraction, which alters the force with which blood is propelled around the circulation. Therefore, an **inotrope** is a drug which increases cardiac contractility. This is achieved through direct action on myocardial cells, by increasing the uptake and utilisation of calcium. It is the level of calcium that affects contractility within the heart (Lisbon, 2003).

Vasoactive drugs affect systemic vascular resistance by altering vessel diameter, resulting in constriction or dilation. Vasoactive drugs have either a **vasopressor** effect, which causes vasoconstriction, or a **vasodilator** effect, which causes vasodilation. Some inotropes also have a vasoactive effect, and vice versa.

How do inotropes and vasoactive agents work?

In order to act, they must have some affinity for adrenergic receptors, which are situated on the myocardial or the cell membranes of the blood vessels. They normally receive the body's natural transmitter substances adrenaline and noradrenaline (hence the term adrenergic receptors). Once the drug has been administered it attaches to and stimulates the appropriate receptor, and a physiological cascade occurs. However, before considering this cascade, make sure you understand the different types of adrenergic receptors and the effect of stimulating them, as shown in Table 6.1. There are three classes of adrenergic receptors, each with two subtypes:

- alpha (α1 and α2)
- beta (β1 and β2)
- dopaminergic (DA1 and DA2).

The different types of receptor are located in different areas of the body, so stimulation brings about different effects as shown in Table 6.1.

Table 6.1 The effects of stimulating selected receptors

Type	Location	Function	Effects of stimulation
α1	Smooth muscle of the peripheral vascular bed	They regulate vascular tone	• Vasoconstriction • Increased blood pressure • Increased preload
α2	Central and peripheral vascular smooth muscle	They inhibit sympathetic nervous system (hence noradrenaline) to the heart and vascular bed	• Vasodilation • Reduced blood pressure • Decreased preload
β1	Myocardium	Modify electrical conduction velocity	• Positive inotropic and chronotropic effects (i.e. increased force and speed of myocardial contraction increases cardiac output and therefore blood pressure) • Increased contractility increases stroke volume (therefore PAP and PAWP can be reduced as congestion in the pulmonary vascular bed eases)
β2	Vascular smooth muscle throughout the body	Maintain vascular tone	• Dilation of smooth muscle • Vasodilation • Reduced afterload
DA1	Central vascular smooth muscle	Maintain vascular tone	• Renal and hepatosplanchnic vasodilation • Reduced SVR • Increased renal blood flow and therefore diuresis
DA2	Renal tubules	Maintain vascular tone	• Reduced noradrenaline release • Inhibition of sympathetic nerve activity • Reduced heart rate • Vasodilation • Reduced SVR • Increased renal blood flow and therefore diuresis

These effects are most commonly mediated by cyclic adenosine 3',5'-monophosphate (cAMP). This chemical is found in muscle cells where it is involved in metabolic and contractile processes. It is produced as the end-product of the cascade, opening slow calcium channels in cardiac and smooth muscle cells and allowing calcium to enter the cell. Stimulation of adrenergic receptors causes release of an enzyme (adenylate cyclase) within the cell. This increases cAMP formation from adenosine triphosphate (ATP). See Fig. 6.1.

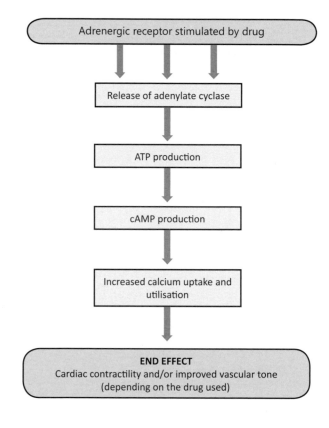

Fig. 6.1 *The effect of stimulating adrenergic receptors.*

The ultimate effect of an administered drug, whether it is an agonist or antagonist, is not only dependent on the agent selected but also on the dose delivered, the characteristics of the receptor, and the response of the individual patient to that drug (Lisbon, 2003).

It should be noted that a patient's actual response to a given dose may be totally different to the anticipated effect; ideally the haemodynamic and pulmonary variables should be monitored with a pulmonary artery flotation catheter or another monitoring device, to help minimise adverse effects.

Inotropic and vasoactive agents act on adrenergic and dopaminergic receptors and are therefore also known as adrenergic and dopaminergic drugs. Adrenergic agents mimic the effects of naturally occurring adrenaline and noradrenaline, thereby simulating the effects of the sympathetic nervous system (in other words, the 'fight or flight response') (Haworth *et al.*, 2004). This is known as a sympathomimetic effect and you will therefore also hear the drugs referred to as sympathomimetic agents.

Special considerations when administering adrenergic agents

1. Hypovolaemia should be corrected *before* administration.

2. NEVER mix with other drugs, particularly alkaline solutions.

3. Adrenergic drugs are irritant (particularly dopamine), so they should be administered via a central line wherever possible. If this is not possible, the irritant drug should be diluted and administered into a large peripheral vein (and the limb should be observed constantly).

4. Continuous monitoring of vital signs should be carried out *while* drug administration is in progress.

5. Vasopressors can cause severe hypoperfusion of the extremities. Observe for signs of skin and/or digit necrosis.

6. If you are unsure of anything or are concerned about anything, *immediately* inform a senior member of staff.

Table 6.2 The effects of drugs specific for different receptor subtypes

Drug	Indications	Actions
Dobutamine	Hypotension Shock	• Acts directly on β1 receptors • Greater inotropic than chronotropic effect ↑ cardiac contractility ↑ cardiac output Also some ↑ heart rate • Modest vasodilation may occur due to ↑ sympathetic tone because of ↑ cardiac output and some β2 stimulation (if large dose used)
Dopamine	Low cardiac output states when inotropic and vasopressor effect required Mainly used in combination with other vasoactive drugs, in a low dose, for its renal effects	• Can activate α, β and DA receptors ↑ • Effects relate to dose: (i) 0.5–3 µg/kg/min: DA1 – renal, mesenteric, coronary and cerebral vasodilation; ↑ renal blood flow; ↑ diuresis DA2 – inhibition of sympathetic neuronal activity (ii) 3–10 µg/kg/min: β activation ↑ cardiac contractility ↑ cardiac output Some ↑ heart rate May also ↑ renal blood flow through ↑ cardiac output (iii) Over 15 µg/kg/min: α activation vasoconstriction ↑ SVR ↑ blood pressure Renal vasoconstriction
Dopexamine	Low cardiac output states Useful for afterload reduction with renal vasocdilation and positive inotropy	• Primarily reduces afterload • Has positive inotropic properties

Drug	Indications	Actions
Dopexamine (cont.)	Main use after major abdominal surgery to increase mesenteric and hepatosplanchnic blood flow (also for renal effects and positive inotropy)	• Stimulates β2 receptors, resulting in peripheral vasodilation, ↑ myocardial contractility and ↑ heart rate • Also stimulates DA receptors to ↑ renal blood flow

Norepinephrine (noradrenaline)	Indications include septic shock with low SVR but ↑ output (warm shock)
	
	CAUTION: monitor for excessive vasoconstriction
		• Naturally occurring catecholamine which acts mainly as a neurotransmitter
		• Primarily a vasoconstrictor (arterial and venous), acting on α receptors
		• Inotropic, acting on β1 receptors
		• Vasoconstriction (except coronary and cerebral vessels which vasodilate, therefore:
		  ↑ preload (PAWP)
		  ↑ afterload (SVR)
		  ↑ venous return
		  BUT ↑ myocardial work and therefore oxygen demand
		• Increased blood pressure may improve renal blood flow and therefore diuresis

Epinephrine (adrenaline)	Useful where myocardial depression and vasodilation co-exist and have not responded to other drugs CAUTION: effects are unpredictable	• Naturally occurring broad-spectrum catecholamine • Mixed ↑ and β effect • Positive inotropic response and a variable degree of vasoconstriction or dilation • Potent cardiac stimulant: ↑ heart rate; ↑ cardiac contractility; ↑ cardiac output • Dysrrhythmogenic • Myocardial oxygen demand and consumption ↑ • In low doses < 1 μg/min causes vasodilation

Consolidation

See pages 125–128 for answers

6.1   What are the main reasons for using inotropic and vasoactive agents?

_____

_____

6.2   What is oxygen delivery to the cell dependent on?

_____

6.3   What is oxygen content of the blood dependent on?

_____

_____

6.4   What is the cardiac output dependent on?

_____

_____

6.5   What three factors must be considered (and acted on where necessary) before or in conjunction with inotropic or vasoactive drug therapy?

_____

_____

_____

6.6 What is an inotropic drug?

_____

6.7 What is the effect of an inotropic drug?

_____

6.8 What effect does calcium have on cardiac muscle cells?

_____

_____

6.9 What effect do vasoactive drugs have?

_____

6.10 What is a vasopressor?

_____

6.11 What is a vasodilator?

_____

6.12 What are adrenergic receptors?

_____

6.13 Name the six types of adrenergic receptor.

_____

6.14 Where are α1 receptors located?

_____

6.15 What is their physiological function?

_____

6.16 What is the effect of their stimulation?

_____

6.17 Where are α2 receptors located?

_____

6.18 What is their physiological function?

_____

6.19 What is the effect of their stimulation?

_____

6.20 Where are β1 receptors located?

_____

6.21 What is their physiological function?

_____

6.22 What is the effect of their stimulation?

_____

6.23   Where are β2 receptors located?

6.24   What is their physiological function?

6.25   What is the effect of their stimulation?

6.26   Where are DA1 receptors located?

6.27   What is their physiological function?

6.28   What is the effect of their stimulation?

6.29   Where are DA2 receptors located?

6.30   What is their physiological function?

6.31   What is the effect of their stimulation?

_____

_____

_____

6.32   Once the drug has attached to the receptor, what do the mechanisms of action involve?

_____

_____

_____

6.33   What does cAMP stand for?

_____

6.34   What is it?

_____

6.35   What effect does cAMP have?

_____

6.36   What does ATP stand for?

_____

6.37   Which enzyme needs to be present for cAMP to be produced from ATP?

6.38   What is notable about the effects of inotropic and vasoactive agents on individual patients?

_____

6.39   By what other names are inotropes and vasoactive drugs known? Why?

_____

_____

_____

6.40   What are the indications for dobutamine administration?

_____

6.41   Which adrenergic receptors does dobutamine stimulate?

_____

6.42   What are the major effects of dobutamine?

_____

_____

_____

6.43   What are the indications for dopamine administration?

_____

_____

6.44   Which adrenergic receptors does dopamine stimulate?

6.45   What are the major effects of dopamine?

6.46   What are the indications for dopexamine administration?

6.47   Which adrenergic receptors does dopexamine stimulate?

6.48   What are the major effects of dopexamine?

6.49   What are the indications for norepinephrine administration?

6.50   Which adrenergic receptors does norepinephrine stimulate?

_____

6.51   What are the major effects of norepinehrine?

_____

_____

_____

6.52   What are the indications for epinephrine administration?

_____

6.53   Which adrenergic receptors does epinephrine stimulate?

_____

6.54   What are the major effects of epinephrine?

_____

_____

_____

6.55   What are the special considerations for administration of adrenergic agents?

_____

_____

_____

Notes

Chapter 7

Putting it all together

Now that the essentials of haemodynamic monitoring have been covered, we can finally put our knowledge to work. You will find full explanations on pages 129–130.

Case study I

Ted is a 48-year-old man who underwent major abdominal surgery for diverticular disease 3 days previously. He was admitted to the intensive care unit in a critical condition. He is very weak, flushed in appearance, sweating profusely, and warm to the touch, although he is complaining of feeling cold and is shivering. His breathing is rapid and shallow and his extremities are cyanosed. He has a weak, rapid pulse and his blood pressure is very low. He is sedated, intubated and ventilated, followed by arterial and PAC insertion. The following results are elicited from Ted's first set of cardiac output studies:

HR 118 b.p.m.	**CVP** 4 mmHg
BP 92/52 mmHg	**CO** 6.60 litre/min
PAP 19/10 mmHg	**CI** 3.89 litre/min/m²
PAWP 7 mmHg	**SVR** 745 dynes

7.1 Give an overview of these results, suggesting a possible diagnosis. What needs to be done to improve Ted's cardiovascular status?

_____

_____

_____

Now consider the following case study and subsequent cardiac output studies. See if you can work out what is going on and what needs to be done. Complete the exercises as you work through the chapter.

Case study II

Cheryl is a 52-year-old woman who underwent abdominal surgery 6 days ago for an intestinal obstruction. Until the second post-operative day, Cheryl had an uneventful recovery. However, early on day 3 she developed a pyrexia of 39.8°C and was very flushed. She felt very unwell, had a severe headache, and felt faint and dizzy. She was commenced on intravenous antibiotics, but her condition worsened over 24 hours. On day 4 she was admitted to the intensive care unit as it was feared she might collapse. For the last 2 days, her respiratory rate was high, up to 38 breaths per minute, but now it has reduced to 12 breaths per minute and she is becoming noticeably cyanosed. She had been passing large amounts of dilute urine but her urine output has now tailed off to less than 30 ml/hour.

She is electively intubated and ventilated and attached to a cardiac monitor. An arterial line is sited and urinary catheter is inserted. She remains pyrexial, with a heart rate of 132 beats per minute and blood pressure of 100/60 mmHg. Her feet and lower legs are becoming mottled. It is decided that further haemodynamic monitoring is necessary, therefore a pulmonary artery catheter is sited to provide a clearer picture of her cardiovascular status. Norepinephrine and dobutamine are commenced.

Consider the cardiac output studies below and write down what you understand from them and the actions that need to be undertaken to improve Cheryl's condition.

Cheryl's first set of cardiac output studies showed:

HR 108 b.p.m.	**CVP** 12 mmHg
BP 102/56 mmHg	**CO** 3.6 litre/min
PAP 31/18 mmHg	**CI** 2.52 litre/min/m²
PAWP 16 mmHg	**SVR** 2096 dynes

7.2 Give an overview of these results and suggest a possible diagnosis. State what action is required and explain why it is necessary.

_____

_____

_____

_____

_____

_____

Cheryl's next studies showed:

HR 112 b.p.m.   **CVP** 6 mmHg
BP 96/57 mmHg   **CO** 3.9 litre/min
PAP 20/10 mmHg   **CI** 2.73 litre/min/m²
PAWP 8 mmHg   **SVR** 1759 dynes

7.3 Give an overview of these results and suggest a possible diagnosis. State what action is required and explain why it is necessary.

_____

_____

_____

_____

_____

_____

The next studies showed:

HR	94 b.p.m.	**CVP**	9 mmHg
BP	118/64 mmHg	**CO**	4.2 litre/min
PAP	26/14 mmHg	**CI**	2.94 litre/min/m²
PAWP	11 mmHg	**SVR**	1450 dynes

7.4 Give an overview of these results and suggest a possible diagnosis. State what action is required and explain why it is necessary.

_____

_____

_____

_____

_____

The next studies showed:

HR	86 b.p.m.	**CVP**	9 mmHg
BP	113/71 mmHg	**CO**	4.30 litre/min
PAP	25/13 mmHg	**CI**	2.96 litre/min/m²
PAWP	11 mmHg	**SVR**	2397 dynes

7.5 Give an overview of these results and suggest a possible diagnosis. State what action is required and explain why it is necessary.

_____

_____

_____

_____

_____

The next studies showed:

HR 84 b.p.m.	**CVP** 12 mmHg
BP 145/63 mmHg	**CO** 6.0 litre/min
PAP 26/16 mmHg	**CI** 4.2 litre/min/m^2
PAWP 14 mmHg	**SVR** 1988 dynes

7.6 Give an overview of these results and suggest a possible diagnosis. State what action is required and explain why it is necessary.

_____

_____

_____

_____

_____

The next studies showed:

HR 82 b.p.m.	**CVP** 12 mmHg
BP 159/78 mmHg	**CO** 4.90 litre/min
PAP 31/16 mmHg	**CI** 3.43 litre/min/m^2
PAWP 14 mmHg	**SVR** 1264 dynes

7.7 Give an overview of these results and suggest a possible diagnosis. State what action is required and explain why it is necessary.

_____

_____

_____

_____

_____

The next studies showed:

HR 86 b.p.m.	**CVP** 11 mmHg
BP 133/67 mmHg	**CO** 4.80 litre/min
PAP 25/15 mmHg	**CI** 3.36 litre/min/m²
PAWP 14 mmHg	**SVR** 1153 dynes

7.8   Give an overview of these results and suggest a possible diagnosis. State what action is required and explain why it is necessary.

_____

_____

_____

_____

_____

The next studies showed:

HR 78 b.p.m.	**CVP** 12 mmHg
BP 123/62 mmHg	**CO** 5.60 litre/min
PAP 24/12 mmHg	**CI** 3.92 litre/min/m²
PAWP 10 mmHg	**SVR** 1076 dynes

7.9   Give an overview of these results and suggest a possible diagnosis. State what action is required and explain why it is necessary.

_____

_____

_____

_____

_____

Clinical samples from a single patient

Collect six consecutive cardiac output study samples from a single patient and record them in the spaces below. For each sample, give an overview of your results, stating what action was taken and whether or not it worked. Discuss your findings with your mentor.

Sample 1

HR		CVP	
BP		CO	
PAP		CI	
PAWP		SVR	

Briefly explain the results, any action that was undertaken and its effect.

_____

_____

_____

Sample 2

HR		CVP	
BP		CO	
PAP		CI	
PAWP		SVR	

Briefly explain the results, any action that was undertaken and its effect.

_____

_____

_____

Sample 3

HR		CVP	
BP		CO	
PAP		CI	
PAWP		SVR	

Briefly explain the results, any action that was undertaken and its effect.

_____

_____

_____

_____

Sample 4

HR		CVP	
BP		CO	
PAP		CI	
PAWP		SVR	

Briefly explain the results, any action that was undertaken and its effect.

_____

_____

_____

_____

Sample 5

HR		CVP	
BP		CO	
PAP		CI	
PAWP		SVR	

Briefly explain the results, any action that was undertaken and its effect.

_____

_____

_____

_____

Sample 6

HR		CVP	
BP		CO	
PAP		CI	
PAWP		SVR	

Briefly explain the results, any action that was undertaken and its effect.

_____

_____

_____

_____

Clinical samples from different patients

Collect six samples from another six patients and analyse them in the same way. Discuss your findings with your mentor.

Patient 1

HR		CVP	
BP		CO	
PAP		CI	
PAWP		SVR	

Briefly explain the results, any action that was undertaken and its effect.

_____

_____

_____

Patient 2

HR		CVP	
BP		CO	
PAP		CI	
PAWP		SVR	

Briefly explain the results, any action that was undertaken and its effect.

_____

_____

_____

Patient 3

HR		CVP	
BP		CO	
PAP		CI	
PAWP		SVR	

Briefly explain the results, any action that was undertaken and its effect.

_____

_____

_____

_____

Patient 4

HR		CVP	
BP		CO	
PAP		CI	
PAWP		SVR	

Briefly explain the results, any action that was undertaken and its effect.

_____

_____

_____

_____

Patient 5

HR		CVP	
BP		CO	
PAP		CI	
PAWP		SVR	

Briefly explain the results, any action that was undertaken and its effect.

_____

_____

_____

Patient 6

HR		CVP	
BP		CO	
PAP		CI	
PAWP		SVR	

Briefly explain the results, any action that was undertaken and its effect.

_____

_____

_____

Congratulations! You've reached the end of this workbook. Now check your answers on pages 129–130 to make sure you have understood everything fully.

Notes

Notes

References

Adam, S. K. and Osborne, S. (2005). *Critical Care Nursing: Science and Practice*. Oxford: Oxford University Press.

Berton, C. and Cholley, B. (2002). Equipment Review: New techniques for cardiac output measurement – oesophageal Doppler, Fick principle using carbon dioxide, and pulse contour analysis. Available at: www.ccforum.com/content/6/3/216 (last accessed January 2009).

Bruck, L., Donofrio, J., Munden, J. and Thompson, G. (eds) (2005). *Anatomy and Physiology Made Incredibly Easy*, 2nd edn. London: Lippincott, Williams and Wilkins.

Chamberlain, N.R. (2004). From systemic inflammatory response syndrome (SIRS) to bacterial sepsis with shock. Available at: http://www.kcom.edu/faculty/chamberlain/website/lectures/lecture/sepsis.htm (last accessed January 2009).

Diehl-Oplinger, L. and Kaminski, M.F. (2004). Choosing the right fluid to counter hypovolaemic shock. *Nursing* **34**(3), 52–54.

Filbin, M.R. and Stapczynski, J.S. (2006). Septic shock. Available at: http://www.emedicine.comemerg/TOPIC533.htm (last accessed January 2009).

Foxall, F. (2008). Arterial Blood Gas Analysis: An Easy Learning Guide. Keswick: M&K Update.

Gonce-Morton, P., Fontaine, D.K., Hudak, C.M. and Gallo, B.M. (2005). *Critical Care Nursing: A Holistic Approach*, 8th edn. London: Lippincott, Williams and Wilkins.

Graham, C. and Parke, T. (2005). Critical care in the emergency department: shock and circulatory support. *Emergency Medical Journal* **22**, 17–21.

Hand, H. (2001). Shock. *Nursing Standard* **15**(48), 45–52.

Haworth, K., Mayer, B.H., Mundon, J., Munson, C., Schaeffer, L. and Wittig, P. (eds) (2007). *Critical Care Nursing Made Incredibly Easy*. London: Lippincott, Williams and Wilkins.

Jansen, J.R.C. (2002). An adequate strategy for the thermodilution technique in patients during mechanical ventilation. *Intensive Care Medicine* **6**, 422.

Janson-Cohen, B. (2005). *Memmler's The Human Body in Health and Disease*, 10th edn. London: Lippincott, Williams and Wilkins.

Jevon, P. and Ewens, B. (eds) (2002). *Monitoring the Critically Ill Patient*, 2nd edn. Oxford: Blackwell Science.

Lisbon, A. (2003). Dopexamine, dobutamine and dopamine increase splanchnic blood flow. Available at: http://www.chestjournal.org/cgi/content/full/123/5_suppl/4605 (last accessed January 2009).

Marieb, E.N. (2006). *Essentials of Human Anatomy and Physiology*, 8th edn. London: Pearson.

Martini, F.H. (2006). *Fundamentals of Anatomy and Physiology*, 7th edn. London: Pearson.

Mattson-Porth, C. (2005). *Pathophysiology: Concepts of Altered Health States*, 7th edn. London: Lippincott, Williams and Wilkins.

Pinsky, M.R. and Payne, D. (eds) (2005). Functional haemodynamic monitoring update. *Intensive Care Medicine* **42**, 188–92.

Pybus, A., Cooper, M. and Bailey, M. (2000). The pulmonary artery catheter. http://www.manbit.com/PAC/chapters/PAC.cfm (last accessed January 2009).

Sharma, S. (2007). Septic shock. Available at: http://www.emedicine.com/MED/topic2101.htm (last accessed January 2009).

Viney, C. (1999). *Nursing the Critically Ill*. London: Bailliere Tindall.

Answers and Teaching Notes

1: Physiological maintenance of blood pressure

1.1 It is the pressure exerted against the arterial walls during the cardiac cycle. Mean arterial pressure is comparable to the perfusion pressure of the aorta, its major branches and major organs throughout the complete cardiac cycle and is therefore representative of the average arterial pressure present in the peripheral circulation.

1.2 The six natural mechanisms for maintaining blood pressure are: maintenance of blood volume; endocrine control; equilibration of cardiac input and output; maintenance of peripheral resistance; the renin–angiotensin system; and the baroreceptor reflex.

1.3 If the fluid volume in the cardiovascular system is reduced, thirst develops to make sure we take in more fluid. At the same time, urine output reduces as a result of ADH production, to conserve fluid within the body (ADH stimulates water reabsorption in the nephron). Conversely, if blood volume increases, thirst is absent and urine output increases to rid the body of excess fluid.

1.4 If blood pressure decreases, the adrenal medullae are stimulated to produce adrenaline and noradrenaline. These increase cardiac contractility, which in turn increases cardiac output. As a result, blood pressure increases.

1.5 As the heart fills with increasing volumes of blood, the myocardium is stretched and the ventricles contract more forcefully.

1.6 Sympathetic nerve impulses maintain a permanent state of partial vasoconstriction which is known as 'sympathetic tone'.

1.7 If there is a decrease in arterial pressure, the juxtaglomerular cells in the kidneys are stimulated to produce renin. Renin is an enzyme that stimulates the production of angiotensin I from inactive angiotensinogen. Angiotensin I stimulates the production of angiotensin-converting enzyme (ACE) from the liver, which converts angiotensin I to angiotensin II. Angiotensin II raises blood pressure by causing an increase in cardiac output and vasoconstriction, stimulating the adrenal cortex to produce aldosterone and bringing about sodium and water retention which also raises blood pressure. ADH is released from the pituitary gland which increases water reabsorption; the thirst centres in the hypothalamus are stimulated to increase fluid consumption.

1.8 Baroreceptors are located in the carotid sinuses, the aortic sinuses and in the wall of the right atrium.

1.9 When blood pressure increases, there is increased baroreceptor activity. This stimulates the cardiac inhibitory centre, reducing sympathetic impulses to the heart, and resulting in two major effects: (i) a decrease in cardiac output due to the inhibition of sympathetic impulses and increasing parasympathetic stimulation; and (ii) widespread peripheral vasodilation due to inhibition of excitatory neurons in the vasomotor centre, resulting in a reduction in blood pressure.

1.10 When blood pressure reduces, baroreceptor output is reduced. This has two major effects: (i) an increase in cardiac output as the cardio-acceleratory centres are stimulated, increasing sympathetic nerve activity to the heart while the cardio-inhibitory centres are inhibited, reducing parasympathetic activity to the heart; and (ii) widespread peripheral vasoconstriction caused by increased sympathetic activity. As a result, blood pressure increases.

1.11 Hypertension increases oxygen demand on the heart because the left ventricle has to maintain an increased workload to maintain adequate tissue perfusion. If the coronary circulation cannot maintain adequate cardiac perfusion, cardiac ischaemia will result. In addition, hypertension places increased stress on the arteriolar walls throughout the body.

1.12 Hypotension results in reduced tissue perfusion and therefore tissue hypoxia and a build-up of waste products.

2: Monitoring blood pressure using an arterial line

2.1 Via the insertion of an arterial line.

2.2 Frequent blood samples for blood gas analysis can be obtained without causing further discomfort to the patient.

2.3 To prevent the backflow of blood along the arterial line and to ensure the patency of the cannula is maintained.

2.4 The radial artery, the brachial artery, the dorsalis pedis and the femoral artery.

2.5 The radial artery.

2.6 It is easy to access, it reduces patient mobility less than other sites, and it is easy to monitor and observe.

2.7 The Allen's test.

2.8 To ensure the collateral circulation to the hand is adequate for maintaining perfusion.

2.9 Occlude the radial and ulnar arteries until the hand blanches, usually for 10–30 seconds. Then release the pressure on the ulnar artery. Colour should return to the hand within 15 seconds. If it does not, use an alternative site.

2.10 Haemorrhage, ischaemia, skin and digit necrosis, thrombosis, air embolism, and infection.

2.11 The pressures within the arteries during the cardiac cycle.

2.12 A is the peak systolic pressure; B is the dicrotic notch; C is the diastolic pressure.

2.13 A reflects the pressure in the arterial system at the peak of systole. B reflects aortic valve closure. C reflects the pressure in the arterial system during diastole and therefore the degree of vasoconstriction.

2.14 The transducer should be calibrated and zero referenced on a regular basis. The transducer should be level with the mid-axillary line (zero reference point) when calibrating the device and when taking recordings. The flush fluid bag must not run dry and the pressure bag must remain at 300 mmHg. If the waveform is dampened or flat, check the patient is not in asystole, then manipulate the arm and flush the line to rectify. There should be no air bubbles in the system.

2.15 Make sure the flush fluid bag does not run dry and the pressure bag remains at 300 mmHg; this will prevent clotting within the cannula and possible thrombosis. Ensure there are no air bubbles in the system this prevents air embolism. Use a transparent dressing at the insertion site, ensure the limb is visible at all times, and replace the dressing when soiled; this enables easy monitoring of the site for infection, tissue necrosis and haemorrhage. Label the insertion site 'arterial line'; this prevents inadvertent drug administration through the line which will cause arterial spasm. Set the monitor alarms to appropriate levels. If the limb is painful, cold, white, or blanches when the line is flushed inform the medical staff; the line can then be removed to prevent perfusion problems. If the cannula appears to have clotted, withdraw blood, then flush through. Remember: NEVER flush a blocked line – ALWAYS withdraw blood before flushing an occluded line.

3: Central venous pressure monitoring

3.1 Right atrial filling pressure, thus venous return, and right ventricular function. It gives an indication of fluid status.

3.2 5–10 cm water or 5–8 mmHg.

3.3 The reading will be higher than normal due to increased intrathoracic pressure caused by positive pressure ventilation.

3.4 The reading will be higher than normal and will correlate with the amount of PEEP.

3.5 For administering large fluid volumes for fluid resuscitation, parenteral nutrition or irritant drugs.

3.6 The subclavian vein, the internal jugular vein and the femoral vein.

3.7 There is a higher risk of infection (because of its position).

3.8 A is right atrial contraction, C is tricuspid valve closure, and V is ventricular contraction.

3.9 Hypovolaemia and/or vasodilation.

3.10 Hypervolaemia and/or vasoconstriction.

3.11 Blood pressure and urine output.

3.12 So that an overall picture can be established.

3.13 Pneumothorax, haemorrhage, haematoma, infection leading to sepsis, air embolism, thrombosis, cardiac arrhythmias, puncture of the vein/atrial/ventricular wall, catheter malposition and catheter tip embolus.

3.14 Strict aseptic technique should be observed during insertion and hands must be thoroughly clean before handling any part of the system (to prevent infection). The flush bag must not run dry and the pressure bag must be at 300 mmHg (to prevent thrombosis). There should be no air bubbles in the system (to prevent air embolism). A transparent dressing must be used at the insertion site, the insertion site must be visible at all times (to permit monitoring for infection and/or haemorrhage). Soiled dressings must be replaced (to prevent infection). Take extra care in patients with cannulation of the femoral artery (to prevent infection). Set the monitor alarms to appropriate levels (to maintain safety).

3.15 As the cannula may have clotted, you would ensure patency by withdrawing blood, then flushing through. NEVER flush a blocked line. ALWAYS withdraw blood before flushing an occluded line.

3.16 As it is likely the catheter tip is in the right ventricle, inform the medical staff so that an X-ray can be taken and the catheter repositioned.

4: Monitoring and maintenance of cardiac output and tissue perfusion

4.1 Thermodilution, transoesophageal echo-Doppler ultrasound, methods using the Fick principle, and arterial pulse contour analysis.

4.2 A catheter for monitoring pressures throughout the heart and cardiovascular system and allowing the measurement of cardiac output by thermodilution. It is inserted via the venous system, by balloon flotation, through the right heart and into the pulmonary circulation.

4.3 The proximal lumen measures CVP. The distal lumen measures pulmonary artery pressure. The balloon port lumen is used to inflate and deflate the latex balloon. The thermistor lumen contains a temperature sensitive wire so that cardiac output can be determined by thermodilution. Extra lumens are used for infusing fluids or drugs or may have a port for pacemaker electrodes or for continuous measurement of mixed venous oxygen saturation.

4.4 Prepare all necessary equipment and maintain asepsis (to ensure all equipment is ready and close by and to prevent infection). Make sure as far as you can that the patient is fully aware of what is going to happen (to gain consent and cooperation). Position the patient on his or her back with the foot of the bed raised (to engorge neck veins to make them easier to locate and to prevent air embolism).

4.5 To observe the pressure traces as the PAC passes through the chambers of the heart (to ensure the PAC is being positioned correctly). To observe the cardiac monitor for arrhythmias (to ensure swift resolution of problems). To monitor vital signs (to ensure swift resolution of problems). To assist the doctor (to ensure a smooth procedure). To give explanations and reassurance to the patient throughout the procedure (to reduce his or her anxiety).

4.6 To zero reference and calibrate equipment when taking over the care of the patient (to ensure readings are accurate). To ensure the PAP trace is visible on the monitor at all times (to check for spontaneous wedging so maintaining patient safety). To observe the insertion site for infection or bleeding (to ensure any problems are dealt with swiftly). To make sure the catheter does not kink (to prevent blockage of the line and ensure readings are accurate). To ensure correct flushing (to prevent blockage of the line).

4.7 Complications on insertion include ventricular arrhythmias, pneumothorax, arterial puncture, air embolism and myocardial perforation. Longer term complications include kinking of the tube (leads to blockage), sepsis, thrombosis, catheter embolus, pulmonary infarction and conduction disturbances.

4.8 CVP, PAP, PAWP, CO, CI, SVR and SVO_2.

4.9 Pulmonary artery pressure.

4.10 20–30/10–20 mmHg.

4.11 Resistance in the pulmonary vascular bed.

4.12 Congestion of blood in the lungs (therefore there is a problem on the left side of the heart, which is not ejecting the stroke volume adequately, leading to back-pressure).

4.13 Pulmonary artery wedge pressure.

4.14 8–15 mmHg.

4.15 Preload.

4.16 The pressure in the left ventricle at the end of diastole (therefore, left ventricular end diastolic pressure = PAWP).

4.17 PAWP also correlates with PAP diastolic pressure.

4.18 Increased preload (the heart would have to contract more forcibly to eject the stroke volume as end diastolic pressure is high).

4.19 By slowly inflating the balloon and watching the monitor until the flattened wedge waveform is visible. The trace is allowed to run for three respiratory cycles (approximately 15 seconds) then the monitor screen is frozen and the balloon is deflated.

4.20 1.5 mL.

4.21 In a branch of the pulmonary artery.

4.22 The pulmonary artery pressure.

4.23 To monitor for spontaneous wedging.

4.24 It is the amount of blood ejected from the left ventricle in 1 minute. Normal value is approximately 5 litres per minute.

4.25 It is calculated by multiplying stroke volume by heart rate: stroke volume (70 mL) × heart rate (72 b.p.m) = 70 × 72 = 5040 mL, which is approximately 5 litres (per minute).

4.26 Inefficient pump action of the heart or pump failure (as seen in cardiogenic shock or the final stage of septic shock).

4.27 A hyperdynamic state (as seen in the warm shock phase of septic shock).

4.28 It is the cardiac output per square metre of body surface area. Normal cardiac index is 2.8–3.6 litres per minute per m².

4.29 It gives an individual body-size related measurement from the patient's specific height and weight (allowing cardiac output values to be compared across different patients).

4.30 It is calculated by dividing the cardiac output by body surface area (in square metres).

4.31 Like low cardiac output, this indicates inefficient pump action of the heart or pump failure (as seen in cardiogenic shock or the final stage of septic shock).

4.32 Like high cardiac output, this indicates a hyperdynamic state (as seen in the warm shock phase of septic shock).

4.33 By thermodilution. A bolus of fluid (usually 10 mL of 5% dextrose) is rapidly injected (within 4 seconds) into the right atrium through the proximal port of the PAC. The temperature change that occurs as the bolus mixes with the stroke volume pumped out of the right ventricle is 'read' downstream by a thermistor in the pulmonary artery. The signal is then transmitted back through the thermistor wires to the cardiac monitor and displayed in litres per minute.

4.34 A minimum of three.

4.35 To effect a temperature change that will be sensed by the thermistor.

4.36 Systemic vascular resistance.

4.37 700–1200.

4.38 Afterload (the amount of resistance that the ventricle has to overcome in order to eject the stroke volume).

4.39 Vasoconstriction.

4.40 Vasodilation.

4.41 SVR that is indexed to body surface area.

4.42 900–1400 dynes.

4.43 The amount of oxygen remaining in the blood at the end of the circulation (after tissue perfusion). It shows the difference between oxygen delivery and oxygen consumption.

4.44 75%.

4.45 Oxygen delivery is reduced, tissue oxygen demand is increased, or both (i.e. there is an imbalance between oxygen supply and demand).

4.46 Oxygen uptake by the tissues is reduced (the most common cause is sepsis when there is a hyperdynamic circulation, because oxygen is available within the circulation but is not taken up appropriately by the tissues).

4.47 There is insufficient oxygen delivery. It needs to be higher than 30% to meet the oxygen requirements of the tissues.

5: The effects of shock

5.1 It is acute circulatory failure with inadequate or inappropriately distributed tissue perfusion which results in generalised cellular hypoxia (more simply, it is inadequate tissue perfusion due to reduced blood flow).

5.2 The tissues will not receive sufficient oxygen or nutrients. Waste products will not be removed. Cellular hypoxia and starvation follow, leading to cell death, organ dysfunction, organ failure and eventually death.

5.3 Reduced tissue perfusion leads to a reduction in venous return and therefore cardiac output; this will lead to low blood pressure, further reducing tissue perfusion. In response, the sympathetic nervous system will stimulate the release of catecholamines, which will cause peripheral vasoconstriction and further reduce tissue perfusion. Reduced tissue perfusion also instigates anaerobic respiration due to hypoxia, the end-product of which is lactic acid. Therefore acidosis develops, leading to myocardial failure. Catecholamines also cause tachycardia and increased myocardial contractility, which increases myocardial oxygen demand while the supply is reduced, leading to myocardial failure. This will lead to multi-organ failure and ultimately death.

5.4 Early shock, middle shock, late shock and fourth-stage shock.

5.5 Increased sympathetic discharge.

5.6 Normal BP with tachycardia, rapid breathing, diaphoresis (sweating), dilated pupils and anxiety.

5.7 Decreased organ perfusion.

5.8 BP reduces (it may be normal), tachycardia, lethargy, disorientation, decreased urine output and cool, clammy skin.

5.9 Failure of compensatory mechanisms.

5.10 Hypotension, a weak thready pulse, an altered conscious state, anuria and skin that is cold to the touch.

5.11 Multiple organ dysfunction syndrome (MODS).

5.12 Loss of function of the major organs (the lungs, kidneys and liver), severe cardiovascular instability, loss of host defences and coagulopathy.

5.13 To provide respiratory support; to maintain/improve circulating volumes; to improve cardiac output and/or vascular tone; to maintain renal function; to eradicate any source of infection.

5.14 Hypovolaemic, obstructive, cardiogenic and distributive.

5.15 Hypovolaemic shock results from loss of circulating volume, even if the heart is pumping adequately. Reduced circulating volume is due to external fluid loss or internal fluid shifts. It results in inadequate tissue perfusion. A reduced oxygen supply to the heart eventually leads to cardiovascular failure, worsening the shock state.

5.16 External haemorrhage, internal haemorrhage (e.g. gastrointestinal bleeding), fractures, major fluid loss (e.g. vomiting, diarrhoea, sweating), renal failure, excessive diuretic use, burns and sepsis.

5.17 Obstructive shock results from an obstruction in the circulation. Venous return is reduced, and therefore cardiac output is reduced and vasoconstriction occurs in an attempt to maintain blood pressure.

5.18 Tension pneumothorax, cardiac tamponade, pulmonary embolism, aortic aneurysm and aortic stenosis.

5.19 Cardiogenic shock results from severe heart failure (pump failure) because the heart is unable to pump efficiently. A low cardiac output leads to low blood pressure, followed by a cascade of physiological effects, with release of adrenaline and aldosterone, causing widespread vasoconstriction. This increases afterload and therefore cardiac work is increased, as is oxygen demand, but oxygen supply is reduced, which ultimately renders the pump action of the heart even more inefficient.

5.20 Myocardial infarction, cardiac surgery, cardiomyopathy, cardiac arrhythmias and valvular disease.

5.21 Distributive shock results from massive peripheral vasodilation, whereby the pressure within the circulation cannot be maintained even though there is an adequate circulating volume. Venous return is reduced as a result of the low pressure, leading to a fall in cardiac output. Compensatory sympathetic nervous activity then causes a rise in cardiac output, but oxygen uptake and delivery is impaired. Fluid shifts into the interstitium from the intravascular space, causing a relative hypovolaemia.

5.22 Systemic infection (i.e. sepsis), anaphylaxis, spinal cord injury (i.e. neurogenic shock) and hypoxia.

5.23 Septic shock.

5.24 Gram negative sepsis (as it is often, but not always, caused by gram-negative bacteria) and endotoxic shock (as it occurs as a result of the body's immune and inflammatory responses to the endotoxins released when the cell wall of bacteria is destroyed).

5.25 Normal symbiotic residents of the gut such as *E. coli*, *Klebsiella* and *Pseudomonas*.

5.26 The inflammatory response leads to increased permeability of blood vessels which allows bacteria into the blood and leads to rapid systemic infection.

5.27 Systemic inflammatory response syndrome (SIRS), sepsis, severe sepsis, and septic shock.

5.28 Temperature alters, usually to above 38°C, but it may reduce to below 36°C. Heart rate rises to more than 90 b.p.m. and respiratory rate increases to over 20 breaths per minute. This causes a decrease in PCO_2 (less than 4.3 kPa) and therefore respiratory alkalosis. The white blood cell count is also raised.

5.29 When SIRS is present and blood culture results are positive (i.e. culture-documented infection).

5.30 When sepsis is present and there is also organ dysfunction with hypotension and/or hypoperfusion abnormalities (may manifest as hypoxia, lactic acidosis, oliguria or acute alteration in mental status, or a combination of these).

5.31 When severe sepsis is present with hypoperfusion abnormalities and hypotension that does not respond to fluid resuscitation.

5.32 Warm (hyperdynamic) shock and cold (hypodynamic) shock.

5.33 There is a high cardiac output, low SVR and low BP as vasodilation occurs (this response makes capillaries more permeable, causing leakage of fluid into the tissues leading to a relative hypovolaemia).

5.34 Fever (leads to diaphoresis and is caused by a substance known as endogenous pyrogen which is released by leucocytes when attacking gram-negative bacteria), increased respiratory rate (leading to loss of water vapour) and profound diuresis (caused by high osmotic load, due to dead bacteria and tissue breakdown).

5.35 With 'creeping' mottling of the legs. DIC is often a complication.

5.36 See Table 5.3 on page 72.

6: The use and effects of inotropic and vasoactive agents

6.1 To maintain adequate tissue perfusion and therefore oxygen delivery in order to meet cellular metabolic requirements.

6.2 Oxygen content of the blood and cardiac output.

6.3 The amount of haemoglobin present in the blood and the degree of arterial oxygen saturation.

6.4 Preload, myocardial contractility and afterload.

6.5 Fluid-load (to optimise cardiac filling pressures), blood products (to increase haemoglobin) and oxygen inhalation or mechanical ventilation (to ensure there is sufficient oxygen in the blood).

6.6 A drug that increases cardiac contractility by direct action on myocardial cells.

6.7 It increases the uptake and utilisation of calcium.

6.8 It affects the contractility of the heart.

6.9 They affect systemic vascular resistance by altering vessel diameter (by causing vasoconstriction or vasodilation).

6.10 A drug that causes vasoconstriction.

6.11 A drug that causes vasodilation.

6.12 Receptors that receive the body's natural transmitter substances adrenaline and noradrenaline

6.13 Alpha 1 and 2 (α1 and α2), beta 1 and 2 (β1 and β2), dopaminergic 1 and 2 (DA1 and DA2).

6.14 In the smooth muscle of the peripheral vascular bed.

6.15 Regulation of vascular tone.

6.16 Vasoconstriction, increased blood pressure and increased preload.

6.17 In central and peripheral vascular smooth muscles.

6.18 Inhibition of the sympathetic nervous system (thus noradrenaline) to the heart and vascular bed.

6.19 Vasodilation, reduced blood pressure and decreased preload.

6.20 In the myocardium.

6.21 Regulate electrical conduction velocity through the myocardium.

6.22 Positive inotropic and chronotropic effects (increase the force and speed of myocardial contraction increasing cardiac output and therefore blood pressure). Can reduce PAP and PAWP by easing congestion (therefore reducing pressures).

6.23 In vascular smooth muscle throughout the body.

6.24 Regulation of vascular tone.

6.25 Dilation of smooth muscle (therefore vasodilation and reduction in afterload).

6.26 In central vascular smooth muscle.

6.27 Regulation of vascular tone.

6.28 Renal and hepatosplanchnic vasodilation (causing a reduction in SVR, increased renal blood flow and therefore diuresis).

6.29 In the renal tubule.

6.30 Regulation of vascular tone.

6.31 They decrease the amount of noradrenaline released and thus inhibit sympathetic nerve activity (causing a reduction in heart rate and vasodilation, leading to a reduction in SVR) and increase renal blood flow (and therefore diuresis).

6.32 Adrenergic receptors are stimulated by the drug, leading to the release of adenylate cyclase which brings about cAMP production from ATP, and then causes increased calcium uptake and utilisation within the cells. The end effect is increased cardiac contractility and/or improved vascular tone, depending on the drug used. This increases blood flow, blood pressure, perfusion and therefore oxygen delivery to the tissues.

6.33 Cyclic adenosine 3',5'-monophosphate.

6.34 A chemical in muscle cells that is involved in both metabolic and contractile processes.

6.35 It opens slow calcium channels in cardiac and smooth muscle cells (allowing calcium to enter).

6.36 Adenosine triphosphate.

6.37 Adenylate cyclase.

6.38 A patient's response to a given agent and dose may be totally different to the anticipated effect.

6.39 Adrenergic and dopaminergic drugs; because they act on both adrenergic and dopaminergic receptors. Sympathomimetic agents; because they mimic the effects of naturally occurring adrenaline and noradrenaline, thereby simulating the effects of the sympathetic nervous system (the sympathomimetic effect).

6.40 Hypotension and/or shock.

6.41 β1 receptors.

6.42 Increased cardiac contractility, cardiac output and heart rate (some). Modest vasodilation due to reduced sympathetic tone (because of increased cardiac output) and some β2 stimulation (with large doses).

6.43 Low cardiac output states requiring inotropic and vasopressor effects. Mainly used in combination with other vasoactive drugs, in low doses, for its renal effects.

6.44 α, β and DA receptors.

6.45 These vary according to the dose: (i) Doses of 0.5–3 μg/kg/min affect DA1 (renal, mesenteric, coronary and cerebral vasodilation; increased renal blood flow and diuresis) and DA2 (inhibition of sympathetic neuronal activity). (ii) Doses of 3–10 μg/kg/min affect β activation (increased cardiac contractility, cardiac output and heart rate; may also increase renal blood flow through increased cardiac output); (iii) Doses above 15 μg/kg/min affect α activation (vasoconstriction, increased SVR and BP and renal vasoconstriction).

6.46 Low cardiac output states. Useful in patients who require afterload reduction with renal vasodilation and positive inotropy. Used mainly in patients after major abdominal surgery to increase mesenteric and hepatosplanchnic blood flow (and for its renal effects and positive inotropy).

6.47 β2 and DA receptors.

6.48 Primarily reduces afterload. Has positive inotropic properties. Stimulates β2 receptors causing peripheral vasodilation, increased myocardial contractility and heart rate. Also stimulates DA receptors (increasing renal blood flow).

6.49 Septic shock with low SVR but high cardiac output (warm shock).

6.50 α1 and β1.

6.51 Primarily vasoconstriction (both arterial and venous, acting on α receptors). Inotropic (acting on β1 receptors) causing increased cardiac output and blood pressure. However, causes vasodilation in coronary and cerebral vessels. Increases preload, PAWP, afterload, SVR and venous return *but* increases myocardial work and therefore oxygen demand. Increased blood pressure may improve renal blood flow and therefore diuresis.

6.52 Co-existing myocardial depression and vasodilation that have not responded to other drugs.

6.53 Mixed α and β effect.

6.54 Positive inotropic response and a variable degree of vasoconstriction or dilation. Potent cardiac stimulant (increases heart rate and cardiac contractility and cardiac output). Dysrhythmogenic (causes conduction disturbances and therefore arrhythmias). Increases myocardial oxygen demand and consumption. In low doses (less than 1μg/minute causes vasodilation. In high doses (over 5 μg/minute) causes vasoconstriction.

6.55 Hypovolaemia should be corrected before administration. NEVER mix with other drugs, particularly alkaline solutions. Adrenergic drugs are irritants (particularly dopamine) and should be administered via a central line. If this is not possible, it should be diluted and administered into a large peripheral vein (and the limb should be observed constantly). Perform continuous vital sign monitoring. Vasopressors can cause severe hypoperfusion of the extremities. If you are unsure or concerned about anything, immediately inform a senior member of staff.

7: Putting it all together

7.1 Ted's cardiac output studies demonstrate that his circulation is failing as the results demonstrate a hyperdynamic circulation (i.e. high CO with low SVR due to vasodilation leading to poor oxygen delivery). In view of his history and symptoms he is in the warm shock phase of septic shock. He requires fluid resuscitation, then drugs to increase cardiac contractility and force of contraction, which will also increase filling pressures and preload. A vasoconstrictor is also required to reduce the SVR.

7.2 HR is high and BP is low, indicating a shocked state. The PAP, PAWP, CVP and SVR are high, indicating fluid overload and/or vasoconstriction. The CO and CI are low, indicating poor cardiac function. In view of Cheryl's history, studies such as this are likely to be caused by the final stage of sepsis (i.e. cold septic shock). She has undergone major gut surgery and developed signs and symptoms of sepsis followed by respiratory depression and cyanosis, low urine output and a mottled appearance to her lower limbs in addition to cardiovascular instability. To improve Cheryl's condition, a cardiac stimulant in the form of an inotrope is required. She is commenced on dobutamine and norepinephrine. These drugs should start to improve her cardiac contractility and therefore increase CO and increase the BP so that her cardiovascular system will not be so sluggish. However, norepinephrine is an alpha stimulant: it causes further vasoconstriction and further increases the SVR. The dose should be reduced a little to reduce vasoconstriction and allow the SVR to return within normal limits. This must be done cautiously to avoid a further drop in BP.

7.3 The BP is low. The PAWP is reducing, as is the SVR, because Cheryl's circulation is dilating. The norepinephrine may be increased so that her circulation does not dilate too quickly and worsen the BP. Dobutamine may be increased to support CO and BP.

7.4 All parameters have improved slightly. Treatment should be continued as per the regimen.

7.5 SVR is increasing and is a cause for concern. The dose of norepinephrine should be lowered to reduce vasoconstriction thereby reducing SVR.

7.6 The SVR has improved slightly but all other parameters have increased. Doses of norepinephrine and dobutamine should be reduced a little to return parameters within normal limits.

7.7   CI is returning to normal although PAP and BP remain high. Norepinephrine and dobutamine should be further reduced to further reduce PAP, BP and SVR.

7.8   These studies show much improvement. Both norepinephrine and dobutamine should be stopped because they are no longer required.

7.9   These studies show further improvement and all parameters are within normal limits. The PAC can now be removed as the patient is over the acute episode of her illness.

7.10   Discuss your findings with your mentor.

7.11   Discuss your findings with your mentor.

N.B. These are suggested actions based upon typical regimens of treatment. Inotropic and vasoactive agents should only be titrated by staff who have undertaken appropriate training and assessment processes and who are deemed competent to do so. Specific, prescribed regimens should always be adhered to.

Index

Index